MW01205826

Fun Things to Do in Retirement

Discover New Passions and Safe Activities that Promote Wellness, Happiness, and Creativity— The Perfect Gift for New Retirees

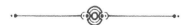

By
F.R. Ferguson

TABLE OF CONTENTS

To you for finally getting to
live your dream retirement.

From a fellow retiree,

F.R. Ferguson

INTRODUCTION

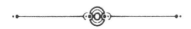

I WAS GETTING TO take my regular Sunday stroll to the doughnut shop when I suddenly felt sad. I was content with my life as it was. Work was good, and my family was happy, but looking out the window as I slipped on my coat, I realized I wasn't satisfied. It wasn't a moment where I felt my heart beating out of my chest or worried about my future. I felt like I had not done enough with my life to feel satisfied. It was nearly time for me to retire, and as I made my way to the store, I decided to look at my retirement plan and figure out a way to bring meaning to my life again. I know it's different for everyone, but there must be more to life than just rushing to work Monday through Friday. It was a depressing feeling, to be honest, but as soon as I got home, I was going to grab a cup of coffee, enjoy a doughnut or two, and figure out my next move.

Retirement doesn't have to be the end of the line. For some people, it is the opportunity to stay home and enjoy an empty nest while they wait for their grandchildren to arrive; for others, it is an opportunity to start over. You don't have to give up on your dreams, either. This is the perfect opportunity to start something new and rekindle a passion for life you may have given up on. Even if you want to spend the rest of your days in the comfort of your home, you can do many different things to occupy your time while keeping fit and maintaining your health.

The government defines retirement as the point to begin claiming your financial benefits. They are no longer responsible for your money, health, or goals. In the early years of our working lives, we are told to save as much as we can to cover our golden years, but what if I told you that your income does not have to end the day you leave the office?

Many people use retirement to chase old dreams and learn new things. You could view it as leaving one type of employment, closing the book on that career, and opening the door to a life of leisure. There are many things to do in retirement, from free college courses and seminars to hobbies and classes. Your life could get even better after you give up your full-time employment and give into living your life to the fullest. Here are the five stages of retirement to look at:

1. Pre-retirement is when you consult with a financial advisor about your money and how you want to invest it. You can attend seminars that help prepare you for your stay at home. You don't have to have an exact plan, but you need a general idea to start taking the first step.

2. The honeymoon stage is where your new life begins. You are finally free of work and can spend some time lounging around the house and enjoying peace. This can be a scary phase if you don't have a plan for the rest of your life, but with the help of this guide, you'll have an idea in no time.

3. The disenchantment stage is where you begin to transform your new life. If you have a vague idea of what you would like to do, then this is the stage where you put that plan into action.

4. The reorientation stage is where you get to know yourself again. You get to live the new life you have planned for yourself and reorient yourself with the ideas you had for your retirement.

5. The stability stage is when you fully accept and acknowledge yourself as a retiree. You have found comfort in the adjustments and are more particular about your life moving forward. You found what you love doing, and you are going for it.

You will know you are ready to retire not just by age but primarily by your remaining love for your career. Initially, it may all seem different and foreign, but you learn to love it as time passes as time passes. There are moments when the colleagues you have turn into lifelong friends, and you live your life intertwined with theirs.

Then, you will get to a phase in your life when you watch your children get older, see them off to college or their respective careers, and feel a bit of emptiness. That feeling may make you wonder if there is more to life, the same way I felt before I retired, and when the moment hits you that you need to settle down and enjoy your life outside your job, you will know. Here is a quick look at what you need to consider:

- Make sure your debt is settled, or you can resolve it with your retirement fund and live comfortably.

- Have a financial plan in place where you can decide on investments before you retire.

- Update your health insurance portfolio.

- If you are below the general retirement age, put a plan to occupy your time and supplement an income part-time as a career change.

Once your debt has been settled, you no longer owe any money on your mortgage, and you have a steady financial plan in place, you'll know it's time. You might be at your complete retirement age requirement or slightly younger, but when your financial status is at a point where you can manage your retirement, and you are ready to settle down, you can begin to look at your options as a retiree.

Chapter 1

EMBRACING THE GREAT OUTDOORS

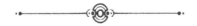

"A walk in nature walks the soul back home."

~ Mary Davis

I T CAN BE CHALLENGING to adjust to a life of quiet when you have spent most of your adult life working and being part of the rat race. The transition from workaholic to casual retiree can be difficult, as I had come to find when I first retired. There were many things to get used to, like not setting the alarm in the morning or racing for that first cup of coffee before I hit the road to miss the traffic, being just a few. Once you enjoy your free time after all your hard work, you get to sit back and enjoy the rewards with more than just a rushed cup of coffee.

My first order was to find something to do other than stand around the kitchen or the backyard, hopelessly trying to figure out the rest of my life. I used to feel like my life no longer had purpose because I wasn't the provider that my family was used to. Yes, I had a great retirement package, but it was different from going out every day and physically being the breadwinner. There was also the issue of not trying to fix things that didn't need fixing so I could keep busy every day, and then I devised a plan. My plan consisted of listing things I have always wanted to do. Things that were easy to access were relatively inexpensive to maintain, and I didn't risk injuring myself if I went overboard with my ideas.

At the top of that list was spending more time outdoors, and since most of my work happened in an office, this was often the one thing I wished I had more time for.

As I stepped outside my home, I couldn't help but feel a sense of liberation. The fresh air, the gentle breeze, and the birds chirping felt so refreshing. It had been a while since I ventured into the great outdoors, and I had almost forgotten how beautiful it was. I decided to take a long walk through the nearby park for inspiration. The lush greenery, the blooming flowers, and the sparkling stream all felt like the holiday I had wanted for many years. I closed my eyes and took a deep breath, savoring the scent of nature. Walking, I noticed how different the world looked outside the concrete jungle. The sky was bluer, the grass was greener, and the sun was brighter, which felt invigorating. I felt a sense of calm wash over me, and I realized how much I had been missing out on. I continued my walk, taking in all the sights and sounds around me. It reminded me how important it was to embrace the great outdoors and spend time in nature while I could.

As a retiree, you can lose sight of all the beautiful things that nature has to offer, and I wanted to show you how some of those things could work for you.

The healing power of nature

Nature has an undeniable healing power. It is one of the most effective ways to reconnect with your inner self and bring peace into your daily life. The smell of fresh plants and colors can uplift your emotions and even bring clarity while adjusting to your new lifestyle. Spending time in nature is a great way to relax and unwind and has been proven to have numerous health benefits. From reducing stress and anxiety to boosting your immune system, there are many reasons why you should make spending time outdoors a regular part of your routine. Whether going for a hike, taking a walk in the park, or simply sitting outside and enjoying the fresh air, there are plenty of ways to get out and reap the benefits of nature. Spending time in nature can have a profound impact on our mental health. Here are some psychological ways nature can help you:

- **Reduce stress:** Studies have shown that spending time in nature can significantly reduce levels of stress hormones in the body, such as cortisol. Even just a short walk in the park can have a calming effect on the mind and body.

- **Increase happiness:** Exposure to nature has increased feelings of happiness and well-being. Being in nature can help us feel more connected to the world.

- **Boost creativity:** Being surrounded by natural beauty can inspire creativity and enhance cognitive function. Studies have shown that spending time in nature can improve problem-solving skills and increase creative thinking.

- **Improve focus:** Nature can be a great way to recharge our mental batteries and improve our ability to focus. Spending time in natural environments is known to improve attention and concentration.

- **Enhance mood:** Simply being in a natural setting can positively impact our mood. Exposure to sunlight, fresh air, and natural beauty can all contribute to a more positive outlook on life.

The great thing about your retirement is that you can learn a new skill while spending time outdoors. With all the extra time, you can choose something simple to master the skill of and take your time to do so. You don't have to pick the most expensive hobby you can find, but rather something small that you can consistently learn to be good at.

Birdwatching

Nature produces the sweetest melodies. Birdwatching, also known as birding, is one of my favorite hobbies—even indoors next to a large window. Just observing your surroundings, even through a window, can have therapeutic effects on your mind. Cognitive alertness is a great benefit of birdwatching. Doing this activity requires focus, which helps the mind to stay active. Listening to nature creates a sense of tranquility, which can help reduce anxiety and depression.

Even if you live in an urban city, you can still do this activity because it is a simple yet affordable activity that you can do without having to do much. If you desire, consider joining birdwatching clubs in your community where you can learn more about the various bird species around you. Each US state has popular birding clubs such as:

- The American Birding Association

- The National Audubon Society

- Birding Pal

You can birdwatch everywhere, and it is a safe, low-impact activity if you have mobility issues. My wife and I became avid birders and desired to embark on a daily observance of a picturesque view of nature right in our backyard. We completed a small backyard project by setting up a birdbath and a feeder to attract the birds. We also planted flower beds to attract hummingbirds and butterflies.

To make your birdwatching ventures more exciting, here are some affordable items to consider:

- Lightweight binoculars that have enough magnification that doesn't cause eye strain

- Scopes if you are an experienced birder

- A resource book to identify the species

Also, consider these tips when it comes to birdwatching:

- Don't wear bright clothing; instead, wear neutral, darker colors

- Wake up early in the morning

- Be patient during these ventures

- Have a notebook to document your experiences

Boating

Many new retirees consider traveling when they first retire. The first options are to buy a plane ticket or hop in the RV for an extended trip, but have you considered boating? The idea of being on a boat doesn't have to include sailing the Great Oceans, but rather a way to enjoy nature while traveling shorter distances with your loved ones. The benefits of boating are endless. Not only is it a fun and exciting activity, but being out on the water is incredibly relaxing and peaceful. In addition to the mental health benefits, boating is also great exercise. As you grow older, you will need to find ways to maintain your physical health, and being on the water can help you practice keeping your balance and coordination.

The sun provides healthy vitamin D, and the change of scenery is an instant mood booster. If you travel to the ocean, you will benefit from constant learning, which can be challenging for new retirees leaving the rat race. Here are a few tips to get you started:

- You need to get adequate training. You won't be able to go onto the water without it. Enrolling with an academy specializing in boats will give you a wider variety. Your license will allow you to sail anywhere and make it legal to be behind the steering wheel of any ship.

- You don't have to buy a boat to go sailing. Peer-to-peer boat sharing allows you to rent a boat the same way you would an Airbnb at a fraction of the cost of buying. You could join a boat club or do a timeshare for boating while deciding if it is a viable investment.

- You must assemble a little kit to make the activity safe. A first aid kit is a must-have. Basic training will help you give peace of mind in case of minor incidents. Other items include lifejackets, flashlights, rope, a personal locator beacon, and a compass.

- You must have a boating registration number or license when sailing, so always keep it in a clean, dry place. If you rent the boat, you must apply the same rule to the paperwork proving you are renting the craft and are trained and fit to go sailing.

- Boat hauling can be a daunting task for beginners. However, it can become a manageable and enjoyable experience with some preparation and practice. Before you begin, ensure your trailer is hitched correctly to your vehicle and your boat is secure on the trailer. Always double-check the tie-downs and ensure that the boat is evenly balanced. Be mindful of your vehicle and trailer's added weight and length when driving. Allow yourself space to brake and turn, and avoid sudden movements. Remember always to follow traffic laws and be considerate of other drivers on the road.

Fishing

We are all familiar with movie scenes where the man goes out fishing all day and only comes home at night with a significant catch. The guy is usually an older fellow who has spent his days working and now enjoys the quiet life along the river, catching dinner for himself and his wife. Fishing is a calm hobby to take up, and it requires patience. If you are in for a life of resting with a beer or two while you wait for your bait to bring in your catch, then this is for you. Fishing is a popular pastime for retirees looking to spend leisurely outdoors. The great thing about fishing is the pride you feel when you land your first big catch. It gives you a sense of purpose again and becomes more than a simple pastime. For retirees looking to cast their line, there is a wide variety between freshwater and saltwater fishing. Some popular destinations for retirees include lakes and rivers in remote areas, where they can enjoy the peacefulness of nature while waiting for a bite. Others prefer to head to the open sea for more challenging fishing experiences. Whatever your preference, fishing is a great way to stay active and enjoy the great outdoors in retirement.

Let's look at a few tips you'll need to get started.

- You want to ensure you have the right fishing gear before you go. Even if you are a beginner, having the right equipment for the type of fishing you'll be doing is crucial. Once you've decided between freshwater and saltwater, you can visit a store and focus on the gear you need for that fishing. Some of the items that every angler should have in their equipment include a fishing rod and reel, fishing line, hooks, and bait. You may need additional gear such as lures, sinkers, bobbers, or a fishing net, which will all come down to the fish you want to catch. A professional opinion goes a long way, so feel free to ask for help at a fishing store if you need clarification.

- To reel in a fish, you must have a good grip on your fishing rod. You will need to focus on keeping the line taut. Now, this might take a bit of practice, so be easy on yourself if you need a few tries before you get the hang of it. Once you feel a tug on the line, start reeling it in slowly but steadily. When you finally get the fish close enough to the shore or boat, use a net or your hands to remove the hook carefully.

- If you decide to catch and release instead of taking your catch home, you must practice doing so carefully. Avoid touching their scales or gills. It's a healthy option for the environment, not to take home every catch but to allow some fish to swim back into the river or ocean.

Regarding fishing safety tips for beginners, you should always be prepared for anything. You first want to remember always to wear a life jacket. Accidents happen quickly; even if you are a strong swimmer, it is better to be safe and well-prepared for an emergency.

You also want to make sure you are familiar with your surroundings. Any hazards like rocks, logs, or other boats can be dangerous if you cannot stop yourself from sailing into them or avoiding them while you're paying attention to your fishing. Bring a friend or family member with you in emergencies and a first aid kit. Even as a skilled angler, it can be rough out on the water, so take someone along that can help prevent danger from occurring.

Hiking

Hiking could be a fun way for you and your spouse or family to connect if you are a new retiree. It gives you the beauty of nature and an opportunity to share a fun activity with your loved ones. It might not be for everyone, but it is an effective way to exercise, get fresh air, and have time to clear your mind after leaving a busy work environment. If you're new to hiking, starting with manageable trails for your fitness level is essential. Look for courses labeled as "easy" or "beginner" and gradually work your way up to more challenging routes. It's also necessary to wear appropriate clothing and footwear, bring plenty of water and snacks, and let someone know your hiking route and estimated return time.

Hiking is one of the best ways to stay active and improve your health and well-being. Some benefits of hiking include improved cardiovascular health, increased muscle strength and endurance, and reduced stress and anxiety. Hiking can also help improve your balance and coordination. Your body begins to slow down as you age, and physical exercise can become strenuous. Hiking can help you remain fit even if you take a simple hiking trail that does not require much climbing.

Let's look at some things you will need to start on your first hiking trail.

- Make sure to check the trail you will take before you go thoroughly. Take a map or a reliable GPS with you so you know where you are going and how to navigate your way off the trail if you get lost.

- Clothing and footgear are essential. If you are going out in warmer clothing, you will need to wear breathable clothing that dries quickly, and your foot gear needs to be an exact yet comfortable fit for grip on rough terrain.

- Take a handbook of all the plants and smaller animals you might encounter on your hike. You want to know what plants to avoid touching and which insects and small animals to look for in your hiking area. A handbook can also guide you in treating your wounds in case of minor injuries.

- Remember to pack the right snacks. Many people don't consider the kind of food they need to take along to make the walk more accessible. Light, protein-based snacks help to aid your body in maintaining its energy levels. Take snacks that are easy to carry, and drink lots of water and fluids that help boost your electrolytes and small protein bars. Or beef jerky that can help you to remain energized without weighing you down.

  Coffee is also an excellent companion. It suppresses hunger on long trails and helps keep you alert, and it has been proven by studies to be one of the best items to carry along with you instead of juice or soda.

Hiking clubs are a great way to start if you don't have anyone to join you. Experienced guides go along on the hike to assist newbies with their experience. It will also help to have someone show you what to do in emergencies. They can talk you through your walk, showing you how to read the signs and use your equipment if you go on an intensive walking trail. Hiking clubs are also a great way to meet new people who have similar interests to yours, which can make the experience fun and light-hearted.

Remember to study the route, the signs you might see, and how to use your essential equipment, like a flashlight and your compass, before you go out, even if you are heading out in a group.

Sightseeing

When you have been bound to your job for 20 or more years, getting out of that mindset of being in an office can be challenging. Some of the most difficult things to do are to get dressed and do nothing but look around the city you live in, with so many beautiful sights to see. Your retirement years are the perfect opportunity to explore your hometown or nearby towns. It can teach about the history of America in a fun way.

Pretending to be a tourist in your city can be fun. There are so many heritage sights to see, and most are free to visit.

Here's what you need to know before you go out and visit these places.

- Search the internet or libraries for historic places in your surrounding area. These hidden gems often tell a story that captivates people and teaches them to appreciate the places where they live. A bit of background history helps to garner excitement about seeing these places, especially if you are not a historian. Note the most profound site and work your way forward from there.

- Decide how you want to visit these sites. Would you like to drive yourself from place to place, or would you like to do a bus tour with other fellow Americans? Going by yourself or with your family can be a fun road trip, but as you age, your friend circle might get smaller, and meeting other people along the way can help you stay in touch with what's happening around you. You might even find a group of friends who want to visit the cities around you and explore parks, farms, or gardens.

- Sightseeing is one of the activities requiring the least research because you're just going out to enjoy the country. It's easy to do because you can get food along the way, you do not need any equipment except a phone and battery charger if you intend to make a long trip, and you can quickly stop off at a motel or an Airbnb if you decide to do an overnight tour.

Some of the best outdoor places to visit are:

- The Grand Canyon

- Yellowstone National Park

- Mount Rushmore

- The National September 11 Museum

You will be out in nature, so you can pack a few snacks in a bag when you go out, but it's an easy activity and less stressful for anyone exploring the outdoors for the first time. Taking a companion with you is always great, but bus tours provide good company if you decide to do it yourself.

Forest bathing

This outdoor gem might seem strange to some, but it can be the most exhilarating experience you have ever had. Forest bathing is a practice that involves immersing oneself in nature, specifically in forests, to improve overall health and well-being. It originated in Japan in the 1980s and has since gained popularity worldwide. Forest bathing is not just about physical exercise but rather about being present in nature and using all of one's senses to connect with the environment. It has been shown to reduce stress, improve mood, boost the immune system, and lower blood pressure.

Forest bathing is a sensory experience focusing on paying attention to your surroundings by actively using all your senses. Experts have said that it doesn't have to happen in a forest specifically, and it can have significant benefits once you incorporate it into your daily life. Spending at least 120 mins a week doing this can significantly impact your mental health, improving your physical health.

To start forest bathing as a beginner, find a quiet and peaceful spot in a nearby forest or wooded area. You can even choose a park if you want to take the safer route and find your feet first. Find a spot to relax and begin by breathing in deeply. Focus your senses on observing the sights, sounds, smells, and textures around you. Take your time and let your mind wander. Give in to the vast silence around you and listen to everything you hear in nature. Focus on clearing your mind for that moment and just being present in that space. Allow the sound and feel of the wind to reset your body while you tune out the rest of the world.

As a beginner, you can start by doing it in your backyard. You can use this to create an open space to be silent and enjoy the sun and birds chirping or a breeze gently blowing across your face. Become comfortable with being outside. Allow yourself to become aware of where you are and how it feels to be outdoors. Once you are at a level where you can venture out into an open space, you can move onto a smaller park until you are comfortable enough to go into a forest.

Safety Tips

Always remember that when you enjoy the outdoors, you must practice safety first. Taking a first aid course can help you in tricky circumstances, so knowing the basics is essential. You could be helping to save someone else along your journey into the great outdoors, so invest in learning how to properly do CPR, bandage or secure your limbs during an injury, or address insect or small animal attacks while you wait for emergency services.

Do thorough research on all the activities that you plan to do. Look at everything you will need to keep yourself and your loved ones safe and how to reach out effectively to emergency services at any given moment. Ensure all your equipment is working or in good condition before you leave home and that you have extra batteries, charging cables, a first aid kit, and safety tools. You might not need all of it at a specific moment, but having it in your car or backpack can give you the peace of mind to enjoy being outdoors.

Sometimes, motivating yourself to go outside can be challenging when you're not in the mood. Getting into the habit of spending time outdoors can be frustrating if you have been sitting behind a desk for a long time. It's not easy to get out of that mindset, and you shouldn't feel guilty if you can't get into enjoying your free time on a whim. These things take time, and there is no rush for you to go from one extreme to the next. You have spent all your time at the office or in a work environment; leaving that takes adjusting.

Many outdoor activities are best done in warmer weather for seniors, which can also play a role. Maybe it's cold or rainy, or you feel lazy. You should spend those days under the covers in front of the TV instead of strolling for fresh air. Finding a friend or a group to join you can make it easier to remain motivated. You may be surprised at how much better you feel after some time outside. Think of the benefits for your physical and mental health. Focus on how much better 20 minutes of fresh air can make you feel if you take the time to clear your mind and just be present in that moment.

Set small goals for yourself and work your way up from there. Your journey into the great outdoors doesn't have to be at an expert level, and once you get the hang of it, you may find yourself naturally wanting to do it. Remember always to be kind to your body when you begin your journey and always to practice safety as you go along.

In the next chapter, we look at ways that you can explore your creative side. It is always great to know what interests you, and with this chapter, you can look at some activities and hobbies that someone could use indoors and outdoors. Knowing my options will be a great source of comfort in filling out my spare time, and knowing what you can do to fill out yours will make your new lifestyle more comfortable. Let's take a look.

Chapter 2

UNLEASHING YOUR INNER ARTIST

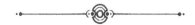

*"Always be on the lookout for the
presence of wonder."*

~ E.B White

W E ARE ALL CREATIVE in some way or another. Finding the one thing we enjoy and making the most out of it takes time. We can all learn new art skills, whether art, sculpting, cooking, or scrapbooking. Retiring is all about having time to enjoy the things you didn't previously have the time for, and becoming an artist might be your thing. It is easy to lose your creativity if you haven't been in a creative environment, and this chapter is all about encouraging you to pursue passions you may have yet to have the time to explore before.

Creativity is not just limited to the arts. It's been scientifically shown that invention can be applied to all walks of life. Medicalnewstoday.com has highlighted studies that show creativity can improve cognitive functions, reduce stress levels, and boost confidence.

Although creativity comes from your genetics and is affected by serotonin and dopamine, it is teachable to most adults and can be matured as a skill. Neurotransmitters influence the cognitive processes in the brain but require you to practice the skill and play around with your newfound creativity to keep it activated. This does not mean you cannot attain creative mastery later in life or improve an existing skill because you're older.

How can art add more color to your life?

Art is a powerful force that can bring color and joy into our daily lives. Something about the infusion of color and patterns activates your brain cells to feel better about life. Art as a method of therapy can take us to another dimension, whether you're looking at a beautiful painting, admiring a sculpture, or even looking at photographs. It inspires us in ways nothing else can. All you need to do is find the right art that appeals to you. When we surround ourselves with art, we are reminded of the beauty in the world and the many views that come from other individuals. Even music has a way of bringing out creativity in us if we make it a part of our environment. Music is often used in therapy to help patients with mental illness or emotional breakdowns. It lifts the mood and encourages people to participate in the activities associated with the music. There is also the bonus of having your stress relieved and your physical health improved if you participate in activities that require dancing or physical movement. Less stress naturally means a healthier body. Exploring your creative side can give you a sense of purpose when you have accomplished or completed a task. It's a win-win for anyone who loves the idea of art and wants to make it a part of their life in retirement.

We need to keep our minds active and engaged as we age, and one way to do this is through being creative. Your problem-solving skills, hand-eye coordination, and memory improve when you engage in your ability to be creative. Even trying something new has its benefits. You need to use your cognitive skills when you try new things, which can strengthen your brain, helping it fight off early signs of dementia or cognitive decline. Reducing anxiety, better sleeping patterns, and clear thinking are all part of keeping the brain healthy. We tend to think outside ourselves when we focus on a task and spend less time worrying about life's daily stressors. This is not to say that being creative is the magic key to youth, but rather an encouraging force that can assist you without requiring too much effort. For adults with chronic illness, the lack of stress can slow down age-related diseases like heart failure, high blood pressure, and other organ damage due to stress.

For empty nesters, it can help to fill up the time that may now seem vast because your daily responsibilities have changed. Not being responsible for children or other adults can leave you with a feeling of emptiness, and finding a creative hobby to occupy your time can boost your confidence and give you a sense of purpose again. Joining group activities will allow you to make new friends and find people with like-minded attitudes. It could be anyone at any age with whom you share similar interests and explore identical art forms. Either way, you eliminate the feeling of loneliness, and you gain a new community that can help you feel valued.

Artistic adventures to attempt: DIY projects

One of the simplest ways to spark your creativity is through home improvement projects. You spend so much time in your home, and being able to turn it into something that you love to look at and spend time in can be a great mood booster, but it will also give you a sense of pride. You can start by turning a simple room into a space to practice your art and perfect your skills.

You'll need to envision the space you want. Look at books or images that come close to your liking. You'll need to start with one wall by hanging a shelf and adding plants and greenery. The benefits of vegetation are highlighted in the first chapter, and bringing it into your home can be an instant mood booster.

You can focus on changing the room's color; there is no need to change the entire room. Start with a small space and work your way forward. The more ideas you have, the easier it will become to get creative. Small projects can help you build confidence to move on to bigger things when comfortable. Learning how to paint the wall correctly or choosing a color you love is an excellent start to understanding how you feel about color and how you feel about painting. Once you're comfortable with the task, you can move on to other projects in your home until you no longer need a guide to help you decide on the space you want to be in.

Woodworking

Woodworking is an excellent hobby for seniors for many reasons. Firstly, it allows seniors to stay active and engaged, essential for maintaining good health and well-being. Secondly, woodworking can be a great way to stimulate the mind, which is especially important as we age. Finally, woodworking is a creative and rewarding pastime that can bring seniors a sense of accomplishment and satisfaction. Knowing you made a piece of furniture or art that you can feel proud of is one way to feel better about how you spend your extra time. Before starting a woodworking project, you'll need a few things. First, you'll need a set of essential woodworking tools such as:

- A saw

- A hammer

- Chisels

- Screwdrivers

- Sandpaper

- Workbench or table to do your projects on

- Safety equipment (glasses, gloves, apron, and breathable masks)

You will need to have good lighting and ventilation in your workspace. This is an exciting pastime, but a few chemicals are involved with your finishing. Once you have the items you need to start, you can look at ideas for making small pieces. Most online apps like Pinterest help you with step-by-step guides through links to other websites, and this can be a great way to start for newbies.

Basic woodworking techniques

Basic woodworking techniques are an excellent help for anyone interested in crafting beautiful objects out of wood. Whether you're a beginner or a seasoned woodworker, there are a few fundamental techniques that you need to master. One of the most basic techniques is cutting. You'll need to know how to use your saw correctly before you start. There are a few options, but a manual saw is an idea for beginners. This helps you to practice controlling your movements and working slowly on your project. Electric saws can be tricky because they move much faster, which can be dangerous for a beginner. Practice cutting smaller pieces so you can get the hang of it first.

Another essential technique is drilling. There are many drills, including hand, power, and drill presses, and they all have their pros and cons. You want to practice drilling holes for small items, and this is where hanging a shelf will come in handy. You can improve your hand-eye coordination and your measuring skills. Drills are powerful tools and can be dangerous if not used correctly, so practice holding them and maintaining your balance before you start on more significant projects.

Sanding is also an essential technique in woodworking. This is how you will begin the finishing of your piece. Each type of sandpaper has its grit level; the higher the grit level, the smoother the finish. Sanding can be done manually, or you can get a power tool that takes the hard work out of getting that smooth finish on your piece. An electric sander takes a lot of the manual labor out of finishing your article and will help you preserve your energy while you work.

Finally, finishing is an essential step in woodworking. A few different types include varnish, oil, and wax, and the use thereof will depend on the piece you are making. I've picked up a few basic woodwork techniques over the years, and the best thing to remember is to measure twice and cut once. Another helpful method is to clamp wood pieces together when gluing to ensure a tight bond. It helps keep the wood in place so it sets in the correct position when you fix it.

Woodworking tips

If you're interested in woodworking, there are a few tips that you should keep in mind to ensure that your projects turn out well. First, always start with quality materials. It's important to use straight wood free from knots and defects. It will make the project more manageable and give you a better finish. Next, take the time to accurately measure so you don't run into trouble later, which can be costly. Remember to practice safety when working with wood. Always wear eye and ear protection and follow all safety guidelines. Asking for help from someone experienced can save you time and money, so look around at local workshops that offer assistance with projects for beginners.

Project ideas

I mentioned that hanging a shelf would be an excellent place to start your DIY projects, so why not begin with a frame? You can make your shelf in any shape or pattern you wish. Online designs for beginners are freely available. This will be a fun project if you want to get used to cutting, drilling, and finishing. A small coffee table is also an excellent starting project because you can often get pre-cut shapes at wood stores. If you want to practice cutting from scratch, a small square coffee table could be the easiest to master. The focus would be to get the joining to work and the lengths and shapes to match, so have fun, but ask for help and remember to practice your safety first.

Safety Tips

When it comes to woodworking, safety should always be a top priority. As listed above, there are a few items you need to add to your list before you start your projects. Here are a few tips to keep you safe while you work:

- Wear the right gear: Always wear safety glasses to protect your eyes from flying debris. Ensure your kit fits you correctly, including safety boots to protect your feet from anything that may fall on the floor. Use earplugs or earmuffs to protect your hearing and the correct size gloves to protect your hands.

- A dust mask can also help prevent inhalation of sawdust or fumes from your finishing products.

- Use the right tools for the right part of the project. Each section you are creating will require a different set of tools that might be different from one another. Using the wrong tool can be dangerous and damage your material or cause injury if you begin to struggle.

- Keep your work area free from clutter and debris. If you have completed a section, throw away the things you do not need or move out of the way so you don't hurt yourself. This will help prevent accidents and injuries.

- Be mindful of your power tools, including your drill and your saw's blade. Work only a little bit of the edge when cutting. Use a push stick or other device to guide the material through the saw.

- Follow instructions to the letter that comes with your tools and equipment. This will help you use them safely and correctly. Remember, safety is the most important thing when it comes to woodworking.

Setting a budget for your projects

Woodworking can be an expensive hobby if you don't set your budget from the start. There are ways to save money without sacrificing quality, but it takes patience and experience. Here are some tips for saving money while woodworking:

- **Use scraps:** Instead of buying new wood for every project, use leftovers from previous projects. You can also ask local woodworkers if they have any scraps they're willing to give away or sell.

- **Buy in bulk:** If you know you'll need a specific type of wood, consider buying it in large quantities to save money.

- **Shop around:** Buy from more than just the first store. Shop around and compare prices to ensure you get the best deal. Ask assistants for advice.

- **Use hand tools:** While power tools can make woodworking more accessible and faster, they can also be expensive. Consider using hand tools instead to save money. Use the power tool option when it gets too hard for you to work with your wood.

- **Make your tools:** Instead of buying expensive devices, make your own. There are many DIY plans available online for making your woodworking tools.

Pottery and ceramics

Pottery and ceramics are great activities for seniors and can be done indoors and outdoors. They provide a fun and creative outlet, promoting dexterity and hand-eye coordination. You can create beautiful pieces of art that they can be proud of and even give as gifts to friends and family. Pottery can be a relaxing and therapeutic experience, and you can include your loved ones in this fun project. Whether a beginner or experienced, there's always something new to learn. It's excellent for your mental health and has a calming effect, which can lower any health risks induced by stress. You can join pottery classes or do a solo activity at a class where you can meet others. Most pottery classes are done in groups, but you don't have to feel obligated to join if you just want to attend a few classes and then go out alone.

What you will need

To get started with pottery, you'll need a few basic supplies. Firstly, you'll need some clay. As a beginner, you can ask someone at a clay store about the best clay to use for starting. You can purchase clay from most art supply stores or online retailers, but a store might be a better option, so you can talk to someone if you need clarification. You'll also need a pottery wheel to shape and mold the clay to your liking. You can try the at-home option of just setting your clay into a shape and letting it bake or use a wheel for more sculpted pieces.

Other essential tools include a set of pottery tools, which will help you carve and shape the clay, and a kiln, used to fire the pottery once it's been shaped and glazed. Some of these items can be bought second-hand, so look at those options first to avoid high costs.

How to get started

Pottery is a unique hobby that can be both relaxing and rewarding. If you're interested in getting started with pottery, here are a few tips to help you get started:

- Choose your tools and materials carefully. You'll need a pottery wheel, clay, and tools like a sponge, wire cutter, and rib. If you do not want to invest in a pottery wheel at first, you can go to a studio where you can use one until you are ready to buy.

- Get to know your materials. Clay comes in different types, each with its properties and uses. Make sure you choose the right style for your project. Feel free to ask for help when selecting your clay.

- Learn the basic techniques. Start with simple techniques like centering, pulling, and shaping. Practice these until you feel comfortable before moving on to more advanced techniques.

- Take a class or workshop. If you're new to pottery, consider taking a class or workshop to learn from an experienced teacher. You'll get hands-on instruction and guidance, which can help develop your skills.

- Don't be too hard on yourself if you don't get it the first few tries. Pottery can be challenging, but it's also gratifying. Keep going even if your first few attempts don't turn out how you hoped. It's an activity that requires patience, so take your time.

Project ideas

When starting, a mug or bowl is two of the easiest things to make. These two items require minimal skill and can familiarize you with your equipment and how to use your materials. These are also fun ways to familiarize yourself with your creativity. You can make something silly and fun and work up to items with a more professional finish. A mug or bowl project is ideal because of the quick timeframe for the clay to set. You can feel proud of your first project that you can own or give to a loved one.

General tips

You want to keep your hands and tools clean while working. This will prevent any unwanted blemishes from showing up on your clay when finished. Try maintaining a consistent moisture level while working on your clay so the finish is nice and smooth. When ready to bake your pottery in the kiln, follow the manufacturing instructions and always wear protective gear like heat-resistant gloves and an apron.

Safety Tips

When working with pottery, it's essential to take safety precautions to prevent accidents. Here are some tips to keep in mind:

- Always wear protective gear, such as gloves and aprons, to avoid cuts or burns from hot clay. The apron will also help to keep your clothing clean.

- Keep your workspace clean and tidy to prevent slips and falls. When you are done with a piece or taking a break, clean the area so you don't accidentally knock into anything to slip.

- Use proper ventilation to avoid inhaling harmful dust or fumes from glazes and other pottery materials. Some of your finishing products might smell strong, so a dust mask can work if you have any underlying health issues.

- Always cut away from your body. Be careful with sharp tools such as knives and wire cutters, and keep them in a safe place when you do not need them.

- Monitor your kiln closely to prevent overheating or fire hazards. If you are working at home, keep an emergency fire extinguisher handy.

Photography

Photographs can be an uplifting reminder of many memories, and what better way to remember moments in your life than by taking the photos yourself? There is something special about picking up a camera and capturing a moment that will last forever. Whether you print it right away or save it for later, knowing you could photograph something special beautifully is something to be proud of.

Photography is also one of the easiest things to master if you have an eye for images or a natural love of art. Many professional photographers started with small things like photographing their families, plants, and animals and later moved on to portraits and landscapes. You could do this, too. All you need is practice and the right equipment.

Some of the benefits of photography are that it improves your observational skills and hand-eye coordination. It's a creative output that lets you capture the world as you see it. There are no right or wrong ways to do it as a hobby. If you want to turn it into something slightly more than just the odd picture being taken, then you can invest in it full-time.

Additionally, photography can help you to see the things around you that you otherwise may have overlooked. It's excellent for relieving stress and relaxing in a quiet space. It can also give a sense of accomplishment as individuals work to improve their skills and capture increasingly stunning photos. Overall, practicing photography has countless benefits. Let's look at how you can turn this into a hobby you will love.

Things you will need

To get started with this hobby, you will need a few essential items to buy brand new or get at a secondhand photography store. Setting your budget is crucial if you are a beginner, so start small and work your way up.

- The first thing you will need is a reliable camera. The kind of camera you choose will depend on the type of images you want to capture. There are plenty of options for every level of photographer, and you can pick up many of these secondhand. Make sure that the camera you select is in complete working order. Using a faulty camera can deter you from wanting to take any more photos, so choose wisely.

- You'll also need memory cards to store your photos and a way to transfer them to your computer. There are also online programs that you can use to keep your images that can help you efficiently access them if your memory cards are total.

- A tripod can help keep your shots steady, especially if taking pictures in low light or using a slow shutter speed. Tripods are also a great help when taking photos outdoors because they allow you to raise your camera to a certain level while you adjust your focus on the object.

- Finally, you'll want to invest in some good lenses. Different lenses will be helpful for different types of photography, so do your research and choose accordingly. There are options where the lenses serve multiple purposes, which might be ideal for a budget-friendly option.

How to get started

Once you have bought your camera and the essential equipment you need, you will want to start practicing. Experiment with different settings on your camera, like lighting and distance, and take photos of things you can easily adjust and move around. You want to work on your indoor and outdoor lighting skills, which is easy to do during the day if you are a beginner. Knowing where the sun is in your photos can impact the results of taking pictures from every angle.

Next, practice taking photos and experimenting with different settings and lighting conditions. Consider taking classes or workshops to improve your skills and learn new techniques. You could even join a class at a studio where a professional photographer can assist you with the settings on your camera until you can set it yourself. Talking to people with similar interests can help you work through some of the more challenging parts of setting up, and it's a great way to network.

Finally, build a portfolio of your best work to gain exposure. Even if it's just a hobby, showing off your results will help boost your confidence and encourage you to keep trying until you get the perfect picture.

Tips for beginners

As a beginner photographer, it can be overwhelming to know where to start. Here are some tips to help you get started:

- Learn the basics of arranging the elements in a photograph. Learn about the rule of thirds, leading lines, and framing, and keep practicing until you feel confident. Take as many of the same photos as you like until you are happy with the result.

- Remember to keep taking plenty of photos. The idea is to get used to how the camera feels in your hand and adjust your hand-eye coordination to get steady shots. Experiment with different settings, angles, and lighting.

- Investing in good equipment makes starting photography easier. You don't have to spend a fortune, but a decent camera and lens can make a big difference in the quality.

- Understand exposure and how much light enters the camera. Learn about aperture, shutter speed, and ISO to control direction. The more you practice, the easier it will be to notice small details.

- Experiment with editing your photos. There are lots of editing software available online that are free and easy to use. Play around with changing the lighting and filters on your images through post-processing. This will give you an idea of the kind of result you would want for your pictures.

Painting and drawing

This is the easiest and most cost-effective hobby you can start with and often needs no skill. There are no rules when it comes to painting, as Van Gogh has proven, and your creativity for how you see your art is endless.

The benefit of drawing is that it improves your fine motor skills and hand-eye coordination. As you age, your muscles may tighten, and the use of your hands may become limited. Drawing helps to keep the function of your hands, wrists, and elbows at peak levels.

If you have hereditary illnesses like arthritis, then drawing can assist with keeping it at bay. It's also a great stress reliever because it forces you to focus on the object you are trying to put onto your paper.

With painting, there are no guidelines at all. You can express yourself in whichever you want; it doesn't have to make sense to anyone but you. The great thing about painting is that it's in the eye of the beholder, and whatever you need to work on can be expressed freely with the stroke of a brush.

Things you will need

To get started with painting, you will need some basic supplies. You can pick them up at a supply store or buy them online. There's no real skill required when you are starting up. The basics will do until you have the hang of it.

These include:

- Paint brushes

- Paint

- Canvas or surface to paint on

- Water bowls

- Some water for cleaning your brushes.

- Depending on the type of painting you are doing, you may also need other materials like palette knives, sponges, or masking tape. This depends on the paint you will use and isn't essential for beginners if you start with water paint.

- An apron to protect your clothing

- An easel to hold up your canvas

- A palette for mixing your colors

Getting started

Make sure your workspace is clean and free of any distractions so you can get as creative as possible. Music can get your mind in the right frame and inspire the painting style you want to work on. Set up your canvas on an easel or a flat surface if you do not have one. Select the colors you like and squeeze small amounts onto a palette.

Dip your paintbrush into the paint and begin painting on the canvas. If you are using watercolor instead of oil, you will need to keep a jar or bowl of water close to rinse your brush in between color selections. Begin with broad strokes to get used to holding your brushes, and work your way to the finer details. There is no right or wrong way to paint because it simply expresses your creativity.

Remember your budget when exploring creative hobbies. For instance, there are many options for painting, especially with the size of the brushes you use, and you can easily get carried away. Buying your canvases in bulk can be a money saver. Art classes also help save on costs if you are still determining the painting you want to create and enjoy an idea of how to express your creativity. Try to work one thing at a time to get the hang of how it feels, and then slowly add more materials as your skill improves.

30-day creative challenge

A great way to start your journey as an artist is to do a 30-day creative challenge. Start by setting a goal or theme for the activities you want to complete. You can include writing poems or making small art pieces. Scrapbooking can be one of the simpler things you do, where you can gather and turn old photos into personal photo albums. Create a schedule for your challenge by making notes of what you plan to do on a calendar and place it somewhere you can easily see it. Your program can include the time you want to do the task and if you want to combine different methods. As you progress through the challenge, try new things and push your limitations through various techniques and mediums.

Include break times for each day, and if you want, you can keep a diary of how far you have come with your tasks to encourage you to continue going. Just remember to have fun while you are doing it. After all, it is a hobby and no longer a job.

In the next chapter, we explore how to discover new passions and how to continue learning. The fulfillment of growth and experiences are topics we dive into extensively. This is to encourage you to continue enjoying your retirement and making the most of the time you have to yourself, so let's get into it.

Chapter 3

DISCOVERING NEW PASSIONS

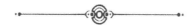

"Retirement is a blank piece of paper. It is the chance to redesign your life into something new and different."

~ Patrick Foley

WITH YOUR RETIREMENT, YOU have more time to look at what you have been passionate about for years. You have the opportunity to explore them. The best part is that you can find new passions and make them your lifestyle as you age gracefully. There is no longer an obligation to be on time for work or corporate ventures, and you can learn to live a new, stress-free life.

Times have changed, and people are retiring much sooner through early retirement-financial independence movements. Although the typical retirement age is 65, some retirees are as young as 40. The opportunity to live life to the fullest is fueled by wanting to do more with your life as soon as possible. All it takes is a step out of your comfort zone to discover things you can enjoy at your leisure.

Look at some interesting facts about the brain and how you can train your brain to explore new passions:

- Your brain is constantly moving and changing. It grows new cells every day, and it's continually evolving its connection.

- When you learn new things, your brain cells reinforce the myelin sheath more efficiently.

- Getting enough sleep helps your memory. Your brain stores the new information you learn while sleeping, so getting enough sleep is essential.

- Your brain finds a way to teach itself old things even when damaged, proving that teaching an old dog new tricks is entirely possible.

- Particular awareness is developed when you do new things regularly. It encourages your hippocampus to grow.

Remember that having a willingness to learn, you will soon discover what your passions are. Learning new hobbies can make all the difference in keeping your mental health in great shape. You only need to apply yourself, and the deed is done—no need to be concerned that you won't get it. With time and patience, it is possible to ignite your passions for something new or old; all it takes is a bit of learning.

The benefits of learning something new are increased mental ability and the fun factor of exercising your body and applying your creativity. We can all change our daily outlook on an old trick in many ways, but learning to redo it is where the excitement lies. The great thing about having extra time on your hands is that there is no rush, and you can find many new ways to make that old thing work. You can explore, research, and find options that work for you in your time. There is no corporate ladder to race up, so the pressure no longer applies to this opportunity.

Learning new things relieves stress and brings joy when you finally get it right. You get a sense of pride from accomplishment that you will only get once you try and apply yourself. Knowing you did it all alone is excellent and might encourage you to continue trying new things.

Ways to cultivate the habit of learning in you

There are many ways to cultivate good habits. Learning can be one of those things, but let's look at some powerful psychological ways to develop new habits that ignite your passions.

- Make a list of your daily routines and build awareness around a specific habit you want to change. A step-by-step guide of what you are most likely to do can help you identify areas needing more attention.

- Changing your habits is a choice; you need to note what you decide to invest your time and energy into.

- Engage in habit stacking, stacking a new practice to something you love doing. For example, if you enjoy running, try doing it after lunch or dinner. It will create a moment of mindfulness that you can turn into a positive habit. Your habit will be to run, and you'll be stacking onto the habit of going for a stroll or running after you've eaten. This will keep you in shape and form a new healthy habit.

- Do things in small doses. Research shows that if you do too much all at once, you may find yourself feeling overwhelmed and quit before you have a chance to get into it. Making a note of things you want to do helps, and as with the 30-day creativity challenge highlighted at the end of Chapter 2, you can add a calendar of habits you want to form and practice daily.

- Remember what your goal is and why you are doing it. This may take a bit of personal insight into your daily routine, but it will open your mind up to the possibility of creating new practices that can benefit you in the long run.

Activities for the lifelong learner in you

In the first two chapters, I have highlighted how online learning can be fantastic for seniors. There are a vast number of things that you can learn, and so many of these online courses are free.

You can start with something simple, like looking at the things you like most and using educational or tutorial websites to inform you of the origin, meaning, and how to incorporate it into your life. Whether you are just researching information or trying to get into a new activity, your options are endless.

Visiting the library or a bookstore that allows you to read the books on the shelves is another great way to relax and learn. Some coffee shops offer books to read while you enjoy a cup of coffee, making it a calming and fun experience. Try reading something that you never thought you would read and try to find an interest in the topic. For example, if you are not a fan of cooking, then read through books that teach you how to start small meals that you can enjoy and present to your family. After making a few smaller meals, you may enjoy cooking and trying bigger ones.

Joining a group specializing in something you enjoy is great for making new friends. Although you may not be in the head space to meet new people, you may find being around different personalities attractive. Bouncing ideas off other people can spark your interest in learning new skills. For example, if you enjoy your quiet time but love making things, then a pottery class or a wine-making course might make things you love feel like a fun activity. Seeing the progress in people on your learning level can be encouraging because you don't feel alone. Having a buddy to make the journey into new learning experiences seem less long encourages people to try new things because their support system increases.

Online learning

Have you ever considered returning to school and taking up that career path you might have put on the back burner? There are a multitude of community colleges that offer courses for seniors at low institutional costs. You can enroll in a part-time course that you attend a few times a week or a daytime system if your time is completely free. There is no need to go out and find a new source of employment. Instead, find something to add to your current lifestyle. With the rage on the internet and all the learning opportunities out there, your options are endless. Some colleges offer tuition waivers for seniors; all you need to do is find one in your state. Here are a few of the courses available:

- Art

- Humanities

- Agriculture

- Computer studies

- Theatre

Each college offers rules for the courses you can apply for and the courses where tuition is free. There are exceptions like law, veterinary studies, dental, and medical, which may have requirements for partaking in these disciplines. Classes can be full or part-time, depending on the dedication level you wish to apply and the course length.

TED talks

Ted Talks can give you perspective. Listening to someone with experience in a particular field and how they navigate their way through things can inspire you to try and fulfill your dreams. Another great thing about Ted Talks is that you can listen to more than one speaker about a topic of interest and get multiple viewpoints. There are TED talks available online, or you can look for TED talks happening in your area at colleges or universities. There is usually a fee for watching live TED talks, but this is the way to go if you want an interactive experience. You can talk to other attendees and get their views on the subject or participate in the Q&A on the day. Most speakers interact with the audience after the talk, which can be another chance to ask questions and get advice on things you need clarity on.

A few Ted Talk topics seniors find valuable involve reconnecting with their inner child. These topics allow seniors to redevelop old skills they may have forgotten or passions they may have left behind.

Here are a few you may find interesting:

- Rediscovering your inner child

- Changes over the years

- Lessons learned in life

- Personal finance and finding your passion

- Self-learning for seniors

These are all relatable topics and can be watched on various online platforms. You can watch Ted Talks from the comfort of your home at a time that suits you. There is no rush to listen to the entire conversation all at once. Take in what you can, and when you have taken the time to understand it, you can return and complete the rest of the talk.

Museums and art galleries

Museums and art galleries offer so much learning. History is one of the subjects that we all tend to set aside as we get older because there is no longer a need to know about old wars or origin stories. If you consider adding art to your list of hobbies, you can learn about an artist or history at a museum or an art gallery. You can ask as many questions as you like and look at all the art and sculptures they have available to gain perspective on the thought behind each piece. The learning opportunities are endless once you build a habit of learning about something you are passionate about. It takes some time to figure out what intrigues you and then move forward. A renowned museum to consider visiting is the Smithsonian. It can be a fun road trip and an excellent way to see all the history and art housed under one massive museum. Nineteen different museums make up this masterpiece of knowledge. It might take more than a day to discover everything they have on display, but it can appeal to the inner child in you as an out-of-town venture. Most students find museum day the best school outing, so why not revisit some of your childhood school trips as a form of learning?

Here are some tools you can use to learn a new skill or explore your passions:

Ebooks and Audiobooks

E-books or audiobooks have taken off in the past decade. Kindle started a revolution in online reading, and with smartphones evolving annually, you can now have your favorite books on your phone to read wherever you are. Listening to a topic while doing an activity can help stimulate your brain because it pushes the brain to focus on multiple things simultaneously. Some enjoy listening to their favorite books while taking a stroll, incorporating exercise into learning. As previously mentioned, this form of habit stacking can take you from an ordinary listener to a super listener and multi-tasker. Think of it as a way to keep your body and mind active with something you like.

We have all seen a scene in a movie where the main character listens to an audiobook while driving to encourage confidence or assertiveness in the workplace. Why not apply this to yourself to apply faith and intensity to the hobbies you want to do? It's effortless to download, and you can race through the chapter at the click of a button without paying attention to the time.

Free ebooks are available online for everyone who wants easy or intuitive listening. You can select it according to the level of learning you want. Here are a few websites you can look at for free ebooks:

- Kindle

- Overdrive

- Blinklist

- Goodreads

You can find these in the Google or Apple app stores. Downloading the app and joining in may be an initial charge, but most content is free and easy to navigate. Reading an eBook is a great way to expand your knowledge and improve your reading skills. The first step is to choose an eBook that interests you and download it onto your device. Once you have the eBook on your device, you can start reading by swiping or tapping through the pages. Taking breaks and resting your eyes to avoid eye strain is essential. Most phones have a blue light-blocking function, and you can turn this on to protect your eyes while reading. You can adjust your device's font size and brightness to make reading more comfortable. As you read more eBooks, you will become more comfortable with the digital format and improve your reading speed and comprehension.

Learning a new language

Learning a new language can be an excellent way for seniors to keep their minds sharp and stay engaged with the world around them. It can be fun if you decide to do it with your partner, but equally satisfying as a solo project. While it can be challenging, many resources are available specifically for seniors. Online courses, language exchange programs, and local classes can all be great options. There are also eBooks available that are easily downloadable from Google or Apple app stores. Finding ways to immerse oneself in the language, such as listening to music or watching films in the target language, helps hear how the words are pronounced. With dedication and persistence, you can successfully learn a new language and enjoy the many benefits that come with it.

Learning any new skill can seem daunting, but it's important to remember that every journey begins with a single step.

One of the best ways to start is by finding resources that work best for you. Stay motivated by setting achievable goals and finding ways to immerse yourself in the language, and don't be afraid to make mistakes. It's meant to be fun, so find a way to enjoy it by incorporating simple phrases into your day.

Several languages are relatively easy to learn for English speakers. The aim is to try remembering small phrases every day that you can practice and say confidently. The more you practice, the easier it becomes to feel confident. Here are a few of the more popular languages that are easy for seniors to learn:

- Spanish has similarities to English and can be easy to master. It's also the most spoken foreign language in the States outside of English. You are bound to find a friend to practice with.

- French is a very passionate language and is both fun and romantic. The easiest way to learn French is by learning the correct pronunciation of luxury brands. There are entertaining YouTube channels that focus on pronunciation. Food that is commonly eaten is also an easy way to work on your pronunciation.

- Italian is a fun language and as captivating as the beautiful country itself. Most people learn to pronounce their Italian words by the name of the places and food, and much like with French, you can use this as a starting point. The grammar is straightforward and may be the most accessible language to master.

Discovering your genealogy and family history

Have you ever been curious about your family's history and where you all come from? It's been a fascinating journey, uncovering stories and connections you never knew existed. When I started researching my genealogy, I found using various online tools and resources helped me. DNA testing and historical records helped a great deal to uncover information, but it allowed me to learn something new. It's incredible to see how far back you can trace your ancestry, and you may even find some surprising connections to famous historical figures.

A deeper understanding of your roots can open your mind to other cultures. What better time to discover where you come from than now?

To research your family tree, gather as much information as possible from your relatives. Ask them about their parents, grandparents, and any other ancestors they know about. As you may know, note where they were born and raised and any travels they may have made before settling in the home. Here are a few things to consider in your search:

- Record their names, birth and death dates, and further important details.

- Search online databases and records for information about your ancestors. Many websites offer free access to census, military, and other vital documents.

- You can also use DNA testing services to discover your ancestry and connect with living relatives.

Remember to visit local libraries and archives to search for documents and records that may not be available online.

- You can also join genealogy groups and attend conferences to learn more about researching your family history and connect with others who share your interests.

Keep careful notes and document your sources as you uncover new information. This will help you stay organized and ensure the accuracy of your findings. You can find fascinating stories and insights about your ancestors and their historical places with patience and persistence.

Ancestry.com and Heritagequest.com are great sources to use. The Census Bureau only dates back to 1940 and requires a subscription to go through the archives. Once you know where to start searching, you can look at library records for dates and events your ancestors or family members may have participated in. For a free search, you can look at Access Genealogy, Allen County Public Library, or Billion Graves.

Tips on discovering your family tree

When researching your family tree, start with what you already know or have. Old family photos and birth or marriage certificates can help find surnames and names for further research. When you have a small information collection, you can use online resources like ancestry websites and archives to dig deeper into your family's history. Verify any information you find and document your sources. Knowing the correct lineage is vital to piece together your family tree. It can also be helpful to join online genealogy communities and connect with others researching their family trees. Remember to be patient and persistent in your research, as uncovering new information can sometimes take time. Please speak to any family members about your information to bring up any memories they may have that can help you find what you are looking for.

Attending lectures and workshops/ local business seminars

Attending lectures as a senior can be both exciting and challenging. On the one hand, you have a wealth of knowledge and personal experience to help you better understand a subject matter. On the other hand, you may need help to keep up with the ever-changing learning methods. Focusing on a class for long periods or keeping up with the class's pace can also be challenging. One way to make the most of your lectures is to come prepared. You must review the material beforehand, take notes, ask questions when you need clarification, and interact with your classmates to make the lecture easier. You will also be required to participate in class activities. Interaction is vital to show your instructor that you are interested and invested in the course. You can also use available resources, like the Internet or the library. Most universities offer tutoring services and study groups, which you can freely join if you prefer one-on-one studying. Then, a study buddy or an instructor can help you to understand the work better.

Even though you are learning a new skill, taking care of yourself will always be essential. Don't push yourself through a course if you cannot get it right the first time. You will have time to catch up. Your physical and mental health must always be maintained to do these activities. Get enough rest, invest in a good diet that supports your journey, and take enough breaks to refocus your energy.

There are excellent opportunities when it comes to attending business seminars. If you choose a workshop on a subject matter, you are familiar with it. You can connect with other like-minded people. Networking helps to work through common problems and allows you to brainstorm with a like-minded companion. Plenty of workshops are available Whether you're interested in technology, marketing, or any other area. Your biggest ally will be research. If you want to maintain your edge in the business world and remain competitive, then having some knowledge of the topic will help. This could also be an opportunity for travel where you can combine a holiday with your learning experience.

Model programs

There is an increasing need to make technology accessible. Understanding how model programs work brings clarity to the latest technological advances and simplifies learning for seniors. Model programs are an ideal way to familiarize yourself with a topic of interest. They are examples of successful initiatives used as guides. These programs have been carefully designed and implemented to address specific issues or challenges and have demonstrated positive outcomes. By studying model programs, you can gain insight into practical strategies and best practices and adapt them to your unique contexts.

You may enjoy going to the library at least once weekly, but with the technology, you can bring the library to the palm of your hand through your smartphone or even your Kindle. There is lots of downloadable information that makes learning these best practices easy. You can store the news on your phone documents if you intend to use them in any of your courses or are attending a seminar where you could use the information. These tips will make attending a local business seminar more pleasant because you'll have background information to help you understand.

Frugalforless.com offers a list of websites with free courses that seniors can use to educate themselves. They are informative, and you can look at various sites under each genre for assistance. It's a comprehensive way to engage with your classmates if you are in similar age groups and makes for excellent study material.

Challenge yourself to learn something new

The brain is a beautiful organ. As I highlighted in chapter two, it can learn at an excessive rate if you allow it to. There is no better time to explore the vast world of the web than through a course, a seminar, or a workshop. Here are a few tips on challenging yourself to learn something new:

- Determine what you want to learn about and research courses, seminars, or workshops that align with your plan. When you have a clear idea of your interests, you can easily engage in research to take the next step.

- Ensure your plan is attainable and challenging enough to push you out of your comfort zone. Be mindful of your expectations and ability to complete the task.

- Create a plan you can easily follow through on. Once you have your goal, create a step-by-step plan to achieve it. Break down your goal into smaller, manageable steps. This will help you to avoid overexerting yourself and to stay organized and focused.

- Sign up for a mentor or a tutor. Finding someone with more knowledge of the subject you wish to embrace can guide your learning journey. Look for someone with experience who is both patient and able to teach you. Sadly, not everyone can train and guide you, but don't get discouraged. Think of other creative ways you can learn.

- Take your time to practice as much as you can. The more you practice, the easier it will become to understand. You can set aside minimal time each day or week to practice your new skill until you build confidence.

- Learning something new can be challenging, and you may experience setbacks. Do not be discouraged. Failure shouldn't be feared, especially when you are learning something new. Embrace failure as an opportunity to increase your learning. You are challenging yourself by reminding yourself of the rewarding experience.

The most important thing to remember on your journey is to be kind to yourself. Leaving a full-time work environment and retiring to a quiet life is an adjustment. There are no shortcuts to experience, and you should embrace it as a part of your life's journey. Asking for help is okay at whatever age you are. You are entitled to feel as youthful as you want during your learning experiences, and your age should never hinder your ability to push through. Focus on how you feel mentally and physically, and take breaks when you feel exhausted or overwhelmed. The great thing about these online courses is that many are free, and you can set the pace.

Join me in the next chapter as we explore the secrets to unlocking longevity. We look at ways to live a healthier lifestyle and ways to promote and nurture your happiness. There is much to live for and many ways to make your retirement time valuable. Head on over to the next chapter with me.

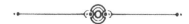

A S A NEW AUTHOR, I am thrilled you are reading this book. This book was created for you in mind to encourage you to explore passions and cultivate hidden talents in your golden retirement years.

Please take 2 minutes to leave an honest review about this book on Amazon. Your review will help others who are considering this book.

If you can, please take a picture of this book and upload it when you submit your review.

Scan the QR code, which will take you directly to Amazon, where you can leave your review. Your review is appreciated.

Chapter 4

UNLOCKING THE SECRETS OF LONGEVITY

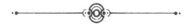

"Life is not merely being alive, but being well."
~ Marcus Valerius Martialis

W HEN YOU FIND YOURSELF in a state of comfort, it can become challenging to unlock new features in your life. Life is valuable and fleeting, and we owe it ourselves to cherish it. Happiness is everyone's dream, but accessing it can have its trials. The most important thing is knowing yourself and finding what works for you. Anyone can achieve this if they are in the right mind to try new things, and the challenge will be to get into that state of mind. As we age, we often feel that spending time with loved ones is the most important thing, but much more can be accomplished. Taking the time to enjoy the simplicity of nature, finding hobbies that you love to engage in, or learning a new skill are all positive ways to bring joy back into your life. Prioritizing yourself and taking care of yourself first should be high on the list of finding your inner happiness and enjoying the journey as you retire. It's vital to prioritize self-care and make time for your happiness.

Over the decades, the life expectancy of individuals has increased thanks to medical advancements and lifestyle changes. Reports of people living past 100 are becoming more common, and many live active lifestyles. They exercise regularly, eat healthy, and spend time with their loved ones. People have begun to cultivate healthier lives to increase their life expectancy. Here are a few starting points you could take a look at:

1. Make time to catch up on your sleep. You need to realize how often you lose sleep before retiring, and now is a great time to make up for that. Sleep promotes good health, and giving your body the rest it needs through a healthy eating plan, some exercise, and rest will be an excellent way to start feeling happier.

2. Focus on being present in the moments that you get to enjoy. Learn to drown out the world and all your concerns in the moments that require enjoyment and focus on how those moments make you feel—being mindful of your emotions and thoughts in joyful moments can't reduce stress levels in your body and increase your mental health.

3. Set healthy boundaries and cultivate positive relationships. This can be hard in a working environment, but having the additional time to nurture relationships with supportive people can help uplift your spirits and make you feel good about yourself. Healthy boundaries will also help you to feel less stressed about responsibilities and tasks that you might not have been comfortable with before and can now limit according to your happiness.

4. Take a moment to relax and have mindless moments.
Whether these include enjoying a TV show you like or having
a cup of coffee in the backyard, take the time to do nothing
but relax and enjoy the sounds, smells, and beauty around
you.

Staying active

We have all heard how a good diet and exercise can improve
the quality of life. Doctors encourage us to go out and move
our limbs and muscles to keep them healthy and functioning.
Our brains also need to remain active as we age, and
maintaining good brain health is as important as maintaining
good physical health. Experts at BetterHelp highlight that
the neurons in the brain die as we age and are irreplaceable.
The fewer neurons, the less our brains can function. This
can slow down our ability to communicate effectively or to
perform physically.

An essential way to promote brain health is to remain
active. Going for a walk, a run, or swimming improves blood
flow and can enhance your brain function. These activities
require minimal thinking, but doing them helps the brain
function better. The release of endorphins helps increase
your feelings; a good mood is always great. Here are some
activities that can help promote a healthier lifestyle:

- Try outdoor exercise instead of going to the gym
  or a class. The fresh air is excellent for your
  lungs, muscles, and bones. The scenery can also be
  incredible for your mood. Try going to a park or
  walking through a nearby walking trail. Hiking is all

the talk these days, and you might enjoy the trails if you're new to this.

- Consider yoga or meditation sessions if you prefer to spend most of your time indoors. Slow, concentrated movements can be good practice, and once you get the hang of it, you can do it mindlessly to relax rather than work out.

- Make time to connect with friends and family in engaging conversations. Mental stimulation through speech is excellent for keeping the brain functioning.

- As highlighted in our previous chapter, a hobby or art form is a solo project you can engage in to stimulate your mind. You can put on some soft music while you work towards completing your task. Better yet, you can get your loved ones to join in with fun activities like a game night. It's a great mood booster and an excellent mental exercise.

Safe, low-impact sports

Taking up a sport when you're older can be challenging. You might struggle to get into something if you haven't been active. The idea, however, is to find something you can easily manage and turn into more than just a pastime but a way of life. Depending on how much exercise you have done before you retired, you might want to ease into something light. If you have spent much time being physically active and can maintain a more strenuous regime, then there is no need to slow down too much. It is always advised to check with your doctor about the current state of your health before taking up a sport and to get an overall check of your body before you engage in new activities that require a lot of movement. Let's look at eight low-impact sports you can do safely and affordably:

1. Walking

Walking is a great way to leave the house and experience nature while working your body into a gentle sweat. There are walking clubs you can join of various skill levels, from experts to beginners, where you can find a group you fit into. If you prefer walking alone, invest in good music or a helpful podcast you can listen to. Remember to invest in good walking shoes that fit well on your feet and cater to your unique needs.

2. Bowling

Bowling is a multifunctional sport you can enjoy, especially as a group. You need to walk and swing a ball at an 8 to 16-pound weight, improving your motor skills and speeding up your metabolism. It's excellent for strengthening your back and chest muscles. It can be done indoors or outdoors and is a perfect way to make new friends or reconnect with old ones.

3. Playing golf

As we all know, seniors often play golf as a leisure activity. You and your companions can play a few rounds on a golf course or practice your swings at a putting range.

4. Dancing

Take up dancing with your partner or join a dance class. It's fun, and rushing through each lesson is unnecessary. You can choose a category that is mindful of your limitations and take time to learn while having fun.

5. Competitive gaming

Competitive gaming, like chess, is excellent for keeping your mind active. You can learn through various online sources if you have never played before. There are online community chess games you can participate in through an organization or be taught by experts who can show you the ropes while you learn. Playing with a partner is fun, but with online gaming becoming so vast, you are bound to gain a competitive edge even in the comfort of your home.

6. Lifting weights

Exercising with hand weights and doing slow and steady reps can help build stronger muscles. When done outdoors, you can benefit from breathing fresh air while you enjoy incredible scenery with the company of others. You can buy a set of weights that suit your fitness level and do it at home with online videos for beginners and seniors. Classes always make it more fun, but you can work up to that when you are more confident.

7. Pilates

Pilates has taken off over the past few years. It has proven to give you the benefits of flexibility and strength training. You get to enjoy a full-body workout using your body weight, and you can do it without any equipment.

8. Chair Yoga

Chair yoga is an easy, low-impact exercise that you can do at home. It's an ancient practice that connects your body and mind through breathing, exercising, meditation, and relaxing poses. Using your chair or the sofa helps anyone with mobility issues or chronic illness. This form of yoga is also ideal if you want to start slowly and find balance. Joint lubrication becomes harder to attain as you age, and chair yoga releases stress and fatigue with gentle movements.

You will need a sturdy chair to sit on to perform the movements. Here is how you can start:

- Sit up straight and allow your spine to extend.

- Take a deep breath. As you exhale, you become rooted in your chair using the lowest part of your spine or tailbone.

- Keep your legs at a 90-degree angle with a little space between your knees, and continue breathing as you roll your shoulders back and use the four corners of your feet to root your lower body onto the ground.

- You can rest your arms beside your body and slowly

bring them up above your head as you continue taking deep, slow breaths.

- Bring your arms down slowly as you exhale, engaging your shoulders and slowly rolling them back with each exhale.

- Take five breaths and slowly begin to fold over your legs with your upper body, allowing your body to rest on your legs and your spine to extend.

- Hold the pose and take five deep breaths. The pose combined with the breathing helps with digestion, massaging your intestines, and relaxing your back muscles.

- Lift your torso back into an upright position slowly when your body feels ready.

These gentle movements activate the muscles slowly while you are in a comfortable position. Chair yoga exercises are preferred over other forms of yoga, especially for seniors who have trouble with mobility.

The most important thing you must always consider is your health and safety. Having free time can lead to trying lots of new things. Consider not jumping from one activity to the other; instead, focus on your ability to see it through based on your health. Your doctor's opinion should always be considered when trying anything that can strain your body and mental health. There would be no point in joining a fitness club, getting into better shape, or having fun if it causes more harm than good. Take into consideration your doctor's opinion and decide on a compromise. If you can do more active, low-contact sports, remember that you only need to do these activities a few days a week, and it shouldn't feel taxing. The idea is to bide your time doing something fun while keeping healthy.

Before you pursue an activity, consider your budget. Fun fitness activities can be costly, whether alone or in a group. Buying equipment and taking classes can also be expensive, so research places in your area that offer free or discount classes for seniors. If you join neighborhood community groups, you might save money as most group members participate for fun, not profit. Walking, running, and swimming groups are accessible at most neighborhood recreation centers like the YMCA.

Challenging your mind

Challenging your mind to remain sharp and functioning at its best is essential. It can become more challenging to keep up with technological advances as we age. Awareness of these changes is necessary, but don't be stressed. A few less demanding ways you can keep training your mind during these years are through board games, puzzles, reading, or new hobbies. There are countless ways to keep your mind engaged.

Breathing exercises

Sleep apnea becomes more common the older we get. Many people who retire from stressful work environments can suffer from breathing difficulties. Hyperventilation is brought on by stress and anxiety, which can cause lung stiffness and make breathing laborious.

Breathing exercises are ideal for anyone, especially if you desire relaxation. These exercises can help you relax while you develop mindfulness and get in touch with your thoughts. This is a perfect time to clear your mind and be mindful of the moment. Your retirement is the time to take care of yourself and your body and live the rest of your life in the best shape possible.

Start your breathing exercise by finding a quiet place. It's essential to be comfortable and to allow your body to feel every breath as you take it. Here are some tips for doing breathing exercises:

- Close your eyes, clear your mind, and relax in the moment. The focus should be on being quiet and mindful of silence and tranquility.

- Take a deep, slow breath, counting to five as you breathe, and then exhale for five counts. Concentrate on the way you feel when you inhale or exhale. Focus on how the air feels entering your lungs and how your body reacts to the deep breaths.

- As your body begins to release the tension through your breathing, relax your limbs and loosen the muscles in your shoulders. Feel your body begin to relax, and your breathing becomes easier.

- Focus on how clear your mind starts to feel with each breath.

Once you become comfortable with these breathing exercises, you can practice them daily as a form of meditation. Consider refocusing your thoughts away from stressors because you must allow your body to rest and relax. With a quiet space and a comfortable position to do these breathing exercises, you might get a different calming effect each time, so it will be ideal to consider doing this daily.

Journaling

Journaling can provide significant relief for all the overwhelming thoughts and feelings you may have. It provides an objective way to separate negative thoughts or worries and gives you a clearer acceptance perspective. Journaling can provide a great understanding of who we are and how we see the world around us. Many people push down their emotions, which can later affect their actions, and journaling allows you to process those thoughts and separate them from reality. It's a way to remember how we feel about moments in our lives and progress with tasks. Seeing your thoughts in black and white can create a clearer picture of your needs. Your emotions may be telling you something, and you can use this opportunity to work through the underlying thoughts you have suppressed. The art of expression is up to the artist, and the contents of journaling are up to the writer.

There are a few key takeaways from starting a journal that can be lots of fun. See it as an opportunity to speak your mind and express your thoughts about your retirement journey, which you can keep entirely to yourself. Journaling is also an excellent opportunity to write about things you cannot easily discuss with others. Many people go to therapy to discuss the disappointments in their lives, and with a journal, you can look at it the same way. Think of it as the therapist who doesn't respond immediately but allows you to slowly reflect on any feelings you may have coming to light in your retirement years. Here are a few things to consider when you start:

- Your journal is personal, so choose a book or format you feel most comfortable with. You can use a beautiful book, pen, or electronic notebook journal. Electronic notebooks are similar to laptops but with less function and are designed to keep notes. What's great about this is that you can store everything, including photos, on this device to explain your feelings in a better way. Holding pictures of moments you treasure with your notes can make the journey more therapeutic.

- Once you have chosen where you want to journal, you must set aside time for journaling. The best way to remain consistent is to select the same time daily. You do not have to journal daily, but journalling simultaneously helps to make it more of a task than just a hobby to pass the time. Early morning journaling helps to clear your head from the day before after getting enough rest. You can enjoy your coffee, think clearly about your feelings, and continue your day when ready. Journaling before bed is also a good idea, but it can be overwhelming right before you get to sleep.

- Now, start writing down whatever you can think of. There is no right or wrong way to do this. It is your thoughts; you can take notes however you like. This is a personal experience; you should enjoy saying exactly how you feel and think and know it is just between you and your journal.

The most common idea behind journaling is remembering what you may forget or keeping notes on your progress. You could be taking up a new hobby that leaves you feeling negative, and journaling can help you understand why. Not all tasks are positive and uplifting. Some may highlight your inadequacies, and you may feel embarrassed or sensitive about them. The trick is to keep writing it down and releasing all those feelings—the health benefits of journaling include strengthening your memory and your brain's receptors. Being mindful of your emotions can also lead to better responses as you age.

You can also use journals to document your travels and new experiences. If your retirement includes planning road trips and visiting historic places, you can start by journaling on those experiences. Other ways to use your journal include documenting your adventures in cooking various dishes, taking up a new hobby like art or woodworking, or spending time outdoors and learning about fresh flowers or plants.

Mind mapping

If you have never heard of mind mapping, you are about to learn something fascinating. Mind mapping is when you organize information using visual techniques. It starts with a diagram in the center of your page or board that branches out. Each branch represents an idea or subtopic extrapolating from a main idea, allowing you to understand your thoughts. Most people use mind mapping to evaluate their ideas and track how each concept can connect to an existing task.

To start mind mapping, you will need a large board or paper to draw your map. Next, you need to focus on your most significant idea and place it in the center of the page. You can leave it free-standing or put it in a box or bubble if you prefer being organized.

The idea or topic you choose needs to be something central that you may want to explore or research. You can create branches (or lines) from the main idea to a subtopic. You will need to develop subtopics that fit under the main idea. This is where you can get creative and use different colors to highlight the importance of each concept. You can even use pictures to make the connection between each thought. Another way you can create the mind map is by using Post-Its to create notes under each sub-topic. You can be as creative as you want. There are no rules.

Self-care

By now, the term self-care should be something you have heard a few times. It is the practice of caring for your mental, emotional, and physical health. A few of the things self-care promotes is engaging in the preparation of self-improvement, whether through relaxing massages or simple meditation. The idea is to reduce stress and anxiety while giving you a sense of well-being and love for yourself.

Following a good eating plan, getting enough exercise, or doing activities that bring you inner peace and calm are all considered forms of self-care. This is an inexpensive way to take care of your mind and body. Meditation helps promote inner peace while improving your body's health and confidence. Consider these four ways to establish a self-care regime :

1. Using technology effectively

Most smartphones have technology that allows you to track your well-being. You can track how many steps you have taken, your weight, your dietary needs, or even your blood pressure. These features help you to understand what changes your body is going through because you can use them as a form of journaling on your smartphone.

Additionally, there are apps you can download that give you a more concise reading on your healthcare journey, like Fabulous Daily Routine Planner, which helps you improve your habits. You can listen to coaching and daily affirmations, do short workouts and breathing exercises, and use the goal tracker to monitor your progress. You can monitor your medication intake and healthcare goals and manage your progress. BetterMe.world is a 30-day weight loss tracking app that can help you track your diet and eating plans. It lists fun ways to change bad eating habits into good ones slowly and gives tips and tricks for boosting your metabolism.

2. Taking care of your body

Take the time to get a pedicure, manicure, or massage. Keeping your outer body in great shape is as important as keeping your mind and inner body healthy. A massage can help with digestive problems and muscle pain and drain your lymphatic system of toxins that can harm your body if left unattended. Acupuncture is a great way to reduce stress and long-term joint pain, and it can help with insomnia. It is also a fantastic tool for postoperative pain, depression, and anxiety.

3. Eating healthier meal options

Take the time to follow a healthier eating plan. Soups and smoothies are easy to make and can be stored for later. They are filled with nutrients and fiber to keep your gut healthy.

Keto works well for anyone with diabetes or who is insulin-resistant. According to Healthline.com, studies have shown that cutting carbs can lead to fewer hunger pains and fewer calories. These studies have also demonstrated that weight loss is more effective without feeling hungry with increased protein intake than higher-carb diets.

As with all diets and eating plans, it is essential to follow the guidance of a healthcare professional before making drastic changes to your diet. Talk to your doctor about your concerns and plans to change your eating habits, and take their advice according to your current state of health.

4. Spending quality time with family and friends

Spending time with family and friends has also proven to increase longevity in seniors. A study conducted by Harvard

Medical School showed that people with a more robust support system who spent more time with family and friends had fewer health concerns, were less likely to succumb to depression, and were less likely to experience cognitive decline.

Showing affection and having social support is proven to have amazing longevity benefits, including a lower risk of dementia, cardiovascular disease, stress, and anxiety. Including your friends and family in your activities or sharing your plans and ideas with loved ones in meaningful ways increases emotional well-being and assists with the motivation to follow through on actions and goals.

Little habits for a healthier you

The first step to better health is to figure out how your current health is doing. A better quality of life starts by seeing your general practitioner to check your blood pressure and sugar levels and to run some mild blood tests to observe kidney and liver function. Also, consider getting a routine eye and hearing examination and seeing a specialist for a routine mammogram or a prostate check. This is the highest form of self-care that you can show yourself. It keeps anything dangerous at bay and gives you the peace of mind you need.

Once clear, you want to take up small habits like drinking more water. Keeping your body hydrated promotes healthy organ function and good digestion. As mentioned before, your diet and exercise routines play a role in the overall health of your mind and body, so make them a daily part of your routine. I have a Sunday routine where I walk to the doughnut shop to enjoy an apple fritter. I make it part of my weekly routine as a personal treat to myself. The walk is calming because it lets me clear my mind, enjoy the outdoors, and have my favorite treat. I started incorporating one healthy meal into my day and increased the meal's healthier contents as I formed better eating habits. If you are used to living on highly processed and sugary food, and the concept of healthier eating is new, starting with one healthy meal daily is ideal.

One of the easiest ways to encourage drinking water and eating healthier as a part of your self-care is to ensure it's always in your peripheral sight. When I began taking better care of myself, I would leave a bottle of water in all the areas of the house where I loved to relax. Seeing the water made me reach out to drink it instead of getting up for a soda or a cup of coffee. Eventually, drinking water became second nature and is now a part of my daily routine.

With food, I found it easier to make a healthy breakfast than to have a more nutritional dinner. Breakfast is the meal that gets you started. If you begin to fuel your body with the good stuff from the beginning of your day, you will add healthier options to your refrigerator and, eventually, your eating plan.

In the next chapter, we will look at how you can begin to enjoy your life and make memories with your family and friends. The first step to enjoying and being productive during retirement is always taking care of yourself first. Once you have the hang of that, you can enjoy your loved ones, too. You will learn how to take the time to invest in fruitful activities with your family and how to strengthen your bond with them.

Chapter 5

MAKING MEMORIES WITH FAMILY & FRIENDS

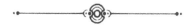

"At the end of your life, you will never regret not having passed one more test, not winning one more verdict, or not closing one more deal. You will regret time not spent with a husband, a friend, a child, or a parent."

~ Barbara Bush

T HE MORE YOU INTERACT with others, the better your chances of remaining healthy. Connection with friends and family is valuable, and spending time with them is a blessing. Studies have shown that socializing reduces stress and anxiety, increases memory function and physical abilities, and uplifts mood. It is also a great way to fight depression, which can occur in later years.

Spending time with family and friends and making memories uplifts the soul. It's the food your mind needs that you can never replace with the things you buy. It doesn't matter what you do as long as you can do it with people who love and support you. Whether you spend an afternoon at home having a cookout or going away on vacation, the moments and special memories you share with your loved ones and close companions can never be replaced. The best part about spending time with others is the laughter, uplifting your spirit, and inspiring creativity. Those memories last a lifetime.

It is essential to make time for the people you love, as it adds to your longevity. Often, people who live well over a hundred attribute their long lives to their love and joy from being around their family and loved ones. Creating strong bonds with reliable people also gives you the confidence to try new things, as you are more likely to do something new with the support of someone with your best interests at heart.

Why are friends and family everything

The people closest to you are the ones who inevitably influence goodness in our lives. They are the ones who support us when we try new things and when we need a shoulder to lean on in difficult times. They stick beside us through the tough times, making the great times more significant. When you need someone to assist you with something challenging, asking someone you can trust is always easier. Knowing that you are surrounded by people with your best interests at heart makes it worth it to keep pushing through troubling times.

Having people to confide in can help anyone struggling to adjust to retirement. Nothing is worse than feeling lonely during their transition from a full-time job to being a stay-at-home retiree. Often, people who retire can feel like the world has been ripped away from them and they no longer have a purpose. Not having a job to go to every day can make anyone feel unwanted or of little to no use to others, but the transition can be more manageable with the right support system. You can talk to someone close to you about loneliness and any feelings that may negatively impact your daily life.

Strengthening bonds with family and friends

A strong bond with family and friends is one of the most vital things in life. As highlighted in previous chapters, these relationships help you to become a better you. In your retirement years, they keep you focused on taking care of yourself, making the most of your time, and giving you a sense of belonging. You can do many things to strengthen these bonds, most of which can be creative and affordable. You don't have to go on a lavish trip to spend time with loved ones. A simple telephone call or dinner with your family can make all the difference in how you feel. All you have to do is make the time to cultivate and nurture those relationships.

It's easy to get caught up in the hustle and bustle of everyday life, but setting time aside and prioritizing your loved ones is essential. While you are home and not busy with any of your hobbies, you can schedule a visit with friends you haven't seen in a while or spend time with your family. During retirement, it begins to feel like everything else is moving on around us, but including your family and friends in your daily life is a start to maintaining those relationships. You can make it a habit to set up a date to have dinner with your family once a month or meet with a friend once a week for a coffee or even an activity.

Be mindful of the time you spend with the people you care about. Being present and paying attention to what they say and what's important to them is as valuable as them paying attention to you. It's a two-way street with lots of benefits. Active listening is one way to show genuine interest in what is going on in their lives, and straightforward communication can help to clarify what is going on in yours. Focus on bringing new topics to the conversation. Meeting with friends shouldn't be just a catch-up of old gossip or baseless chats. Make it enjoyable by telling your friends about new things you've done and inviting them to join you. You would be pleasantly surprised how many friends or loved ones might like to participate in some of your activities.

Always show appreciation for the people who make time for you. Let them know that you value the time they are taking to spend with you, and let them know how much they mean to you. There is no shame in being honest about needing people; that is what most people need to hear. They need to know that they are valued and essential to you. This can be as easy as a text from time to time to remind someone you love that you are thinking about them and that you hope they are doing well. Acknowledging their achievements can also go a long way in building meaningful relationships.

Remember that there are no perfect relationships. No one is perfect, and we are all flawed as humans. Give your family and loved ones the space to be themselves and feel safe to engage with you despite any flaws they may have. Learn to be forgiving and accepting, and be compassionate. Open communication can be the key to resolving conflict or issues that may bother you. Communication helps create a safe space and shows an effort to determine and maintain relationships.

How to organize a family get-together

Organizing a family get-together can be a fun and rewarding experience. Here are six tips to help you plan a successful event:

1. Plan your event. Give everyone enough time to plan and set their schedules. Choose a central place for everyone to go to if you are not having the get-together at your home. Think of how many people you want to invite and if the space can accommodate everyone comfortably. The more, the merrier, as long as everyone is at ease, able to attend, and comfortable when they arrive.

2. Identify the location of the event. Where you decide to get together depends on the weather, and you want to cater to both sun and rain. Preparing for anything makes all the difference and can make even the worst weather enjoyable if you have a plan. You want your guests to be comfortable and safe, so think of places that cater to all weather conditions. If you are organizing a camping or day trip to the park or beach, consider what's needed and be prepared for essential items like flashlights, first aid kits, ice coolers, food, and utensils.

3. Prepare a menu. Decide on what you want to serve your guests on the day. The menu you choose can be light or a full 4-course meal, depending on the event's theme. Ensure you cater to everyone's dietary requirements, whether having a barbeque, potluck, or a sit-down. You also want to have the right catering equipment. If you're having a fun outdoor event, consider things you can throw away to make the cleaning easier. Consider getting extra glasses and bowls to match each course for a sit-down.

4. Plan activities. If your get-together is during the day and you plan on spending time outside, you need to have activities for everyone to do. Not everyone will want to run around playing a sport or participating in board games, but being prepared for that is essential in making the time together memorable. Depending on your family members' age range and interests, plan some games or activities to keep everyone entertained.

5. Send invitations. Whether it be a text or call, provide an invitation to invite your guests formally. When you send out your invitations, add an RSVP date and number so guests can let you know if they can attend. The RSVP section will help you to cater to everyone and to ensure that you have identified persons with special dietary needs. Be clear about the location, the time, and the date you will be having your get-together. Send out the invitations at least a month before the event to give everyone enough time to organize themselves in case they need to travel.

6. Be organized and prepared for smaller, intimate gatherings at home. If your family and friends come to your home, ensure you have prepared for everything. Ensure everything you need is set up and ready before your guest arrives. You want to avoid running around for last-minute items so that you can spend more time enjoying your company.

Remember, this is meant to be a joyous time with your family, and the aim is to have fun. Don't be too overly concerned if things don't go as planned. Take the load off and just be present. Be yourself around the people who matter the most to you. The idea is to be there with them and engage in meaningful bonding. The best part is that you can make lots of memories. If you have taken up amateur photography as a hobby, this is a great time to practice what you've learned. You can store those memories or use them as an opportunity to gift your family with fun photos of your time together.

Host a Potluck for family and loved ones

Potluck gatherings have become the new way to enjoy food without the hassle of going to a restaurant. It is a dinner where everyone attending brings their favorite dish to share with everyone else attending. It's an excellent way to try new foods while enjoying the company of others. Some potluck gatherings may have a theme where the food incorporates other cultures, and you could even dress up to make it more interesting.

Potlucks are informal dinner parties held at someone's home, rental space, or community center. It can be done with family or the community around you to make it more fun. It's an affordable way to get family and friends to spend time together while learning about other food types they may not ordinarily eat. Hosting a potluck is a unique and creative way to unite people, and it's easy to organize when you have all the basics under wraps. Let's look at how to manage and enjoy a successful potluck:

1. Set a date and send out your invites. If you have it at a community center, you should put up posters with a contact number or email address so participants can tell you what they will bring and if they can attend. You do not want a few of the same dishes, so list everyone coming and the food they plan to bring.

2. Do your research. If you are having a themed event, research dishes that go together with the theme to give your guests some ideas. Make sure to divide the starters, mains, and deserts evenly so you don't end up with ten deserts and only three main meals. Consider thinking of drinks, so let your guests know to bring something along if you are not catering to the drinks yourself. If there are any guests with allergies, you need to inform everyone on the list so they know to avoid adding certain ingredients to every meal.

3. Be prepared. As the host, you must provide basics like ice, cups, plates, and napkins. If the plates and utensils you use are recyclable, have the recycling and waste bins in sight so guests know where to dispose of their trash when they finish their meals. It makes it easier to keep things under control and less messy.

4. Organize serving and seating tables. You want enough space for everyone to lay out their dishes. The room must be big enough for the serving table to hold most of the dishes without looking cluttered. Ensure each dish has its designated serving utensil in case guests have allergies. For easy clean up, consider providing wet wipes and dishcloths for easy cleaning and wiping of dishes so that your guests can take them home.

5. Get creative and have fun. If you have a theme for the evening, think of adding decor or asking everyone to come dressed up as the theme. This will make the evening more fun. For example, if the theme is Mexican, add some margaritas as welcome drinks or play Mexican music in the background to add to the ambiance.

Potluck etiquette

The most vital thing to consider is what others may want to eat. Some may have dietary restrictions due to health issues or simply because they don't eat meat or other food types. As the host, you must ask your guests for these details so it's a fun night for everyone attending. Ask your guests to label their dishes, and as a fun idea, ask them to add sauces or sides to complement the food they are serving. Always allow your guests to serve themselves before you do. As the host, your hospitality will ensure all the guests are comfortable and have everything they need, like utensils, cups, and proper seating.

How to host a modern potluck

1. Think of the food you want everyone to bring to your potluck. Would the meals be healthy or international? Are they tapas-style meals or full-course meals? This can make it easier to set up a menu and make it convenient for guests to decide what they would like to bring. If you want to avoid giving your guests a menu to choose from, set several starters, mains, and deserts so the courses are even. For example, if you have twenty guests coming, you can ask five people to bring mains, five to bring starters, five to bring snack bowls, and five to get desserts.

2. Consider assigning each guest a dish if your event has no theme. You want to avoid having four guests bring lasagne, so ask each guest to get a specific meal from a list. This will also make it easier to track your meals and how many more you'll need. Ask guests to bring meals that serve enough guests in case everyone decides to eat from one specific dish.

3. Plan your menu accordingly. Do as much research as possible and give guests options on the meals they could bring. Most people might need a clearer idea of what to contribute, so give them examples to make it easier to get excited about attending.

4. Serving utensils like spoons, tongs, and forks are sometimes on the list of things people bring along, so make sure you have enough. You can add condiments and extra spices like salt, pepper, garlic, or chili for anyone who might like a different flavor for their meal. If any of your meals include pizza or pasta, then a side serving of parmesan will make a welcomed addition to your condiments.

5. If your venue doesn't have a bar, you could make a drink station instead. This separates the drinks from the food and allocates a designated area where guests can fill their glasses and collect their cups. Include water pitchers and soft drinks for anyone who might not be consuming any alcohol or just as an added treat for guests taking a break in between meals.

6. Provide guests with utensils, cups, and plates in case someone forgets to bring them. You can ask your guests to bring their items, but consider that someone may forget to bring the promised items.

7. Add decor to the venue. The set gives an authentic feel to your chosen theme, making for fun conversation. It's a way for people to start talking, especially if they wear a costume that matches the night's theme. Scented candles, flowers, and music add to the evening, so make that a part of your list when you decorate.

Potlucks are a fun way to unite people, and there should be no pressure from the host or guests in the evening. You want to have a great time socializing, so keep your checklist handy before the evening to ensure you have everything you need and don't run out of anything on the night of your dinner party. It's always handy to have extras.

Building new bonds

You might find it harder to make new friends and build new bonds with strangers. It is essential to keep good relationships, but making new friends can open you up to a world of things you wouldn't normally engage in. Your old circle might enjoy a quieter life, but new friends can help you find new adventures. This is imperative to living a longer life. You will need new things to keep you excited about life; sharing that with people with mutual interests helps. You must show genuine interest in the people you are getting to know. Taking an interest in their journey in life and the things that matter to them shows that you are looking to stick around rather than pass the time. You have to make time to hang out with others in a setting that interests them as much as you and sometimes let them decide on your plans when you spend time together.

Activities that encourage social interactions

You can participate in many activities to help you socially interact with others. The best way to meet new people is through groups or clubs that offer activities aligning with your interests. You can join a book club, a cooking class, or even a sporting club to meet or socialize with others. Not only will you have the opportunity to connect with new people, but you can use this as a chance to reconnect with old friends who share similar passions. These clubs or groups allow you to catch up with anyone you may not have seen in a while due to work obligations, and you can both learn new skills or rekindle passions.

Another fun thing you can consider is watching your favorite band or attending an art show. Live events are always fun, and there are many things to see. Concerts allow you to reconnect through music, and festivals will enable you to interact with others while you enjoy the vibe and the music. These events bring people together and are designed to help people feel uplifted and happy. It allows you to meet like-minded people or spend time with both old or new friends or perhaps acquaintances. There are also low-impact sports like bowling or indoor golf to help you stay fit while you socialize, and the competitive design of these activities makes for a friendly battle amongst teams if you participate in groups.

Volunteering

If you have ever been passionate about a charity or a cause, your retirement is the ideal time to pursue volunteering opportunities. Many non-profit organizations need help. If you take a friend along, you can make it a social event. Not only will you be doing good for the community or cause, but you will also be spending time with your friends. Consider volunteering for your local community projects or researching other non-profit organizations that may need assistance. This is a feel-good effort that can be fun and rewarding. Start with small projects like cleaning up around the neighborhood or restoring a community center that may need new paint or extra facilities. This also gives you a chance to practice some of your art skills like painting or woodwork, where you can contribute to the project by giving them some of your work as a gift.

Social media is a powerful tool that you can use to connect to friends and family, and if you still need to venture into becoming tech-savvy, then this is a good start. Online forums such as Facebook (now Meta) and Nextdoor are very popular social media platforms where users can connect with these charities. Charities and not-for-profits have social media accounts where you can research and be informed about their purpose and mission. Before you donate money to any organization, be sure to do your due diligence in researching these groups, their causes, and their intentions. Also, consider their history and practices and decide whether they closely align with your values and beliefs. If you do not have anyone to go with, you can always connect through these platforms with like-minded people who also believe in the causes you do. This may not be as personal as meeting people in real life, but social media can help provide a sense of connection with others who share your views and interests.

Volunteering is a way to contribute back to your community. You can make a difference in the lives of others simply by being present and mindful of their needs and circumstances. The endless rewards can boost your confidence in stepping out of your comfort zone and making it a regular part of your life. Helping others in community projects or volunteering at shelters, soup kitchens, or animal shelters can give you the meaning you seek. If volunteering sounds like something you would like to consider, then you may want to consider these three easy steps to make your experience a successful one:

1. Figure out what you like doing and what causes mean the most to you. Identifying your passions will make connecting to organizations or charities of like-minded interests easier. Once you have narrowed down the ones you want to explore, focus on starting with the more convenient one and working your way down the list.

2. Use the internet to find organizations in your area that need volunteers and find out if they allow seniors to participate. Some causes require manual labor, which might not be ideal for you. Contact the organization about your concerns and ask about the requirements or training programs required to be completed before being allowed to volunteer.

3. Spend time preparing for your volunteering role. If you need to attend a training session or two, sign up for an orientation. This will give you an idea of the program or cause and allow you to ask questions and get direct answers. Not all organizations have orientation classes for their volunteers, but it will serve you best to sign up for the ones that do. That way, you can learn about the requirements and how to succeed in your volunteering role.

As with everything, ensuring your safety and well-being is essential. Working in a specific environment may seem like a good idea, but it might not be suitable to pursue if it causes you to feel any form of stress. Volunteering is a great way to make new friends and meet new people, but some volunteering roles are more challenging than others. Do not feel bad if you do not meet the requirements or if a cause you love doesn't suit your well-being needs. There will be other ways to contribute, so do your research and find out what will suit you best.

Social media interactions

If you have not spent much time on the internet lately and want to join the world of social media, then this is for you. New platforms are popping up, and many of them can be complex, but for a beginner, the best ones are the ones your loved ones use. Choosing a platform where you can connect with your loved ones first will allow you to get the hang of using the apps before you venture out into the rest of the world of social media. You can practice using the instant messaging features to send quick messages to your loved ones. These apps can also reconnect you with friends from high school or college and give you a chance to rebuild lost relationships. You can meet new people in fun groups, and you can get updates on fun activities that are happening around you. Some theaters and studios use social media to advertise events they host and allow you to sign up for them via the platform. You can even share those events with your friends on the platform so they get the information, too.

Some groups on social media platforms also advertise events, courses, and classes they host to promote their businesses, like cooking, art, or music. You can find people with similar interests in the likes and comments for events. The platform has capabilities for letting you know about events other people in your community are interested in attending, which makes connecting with others easier.

In the next chapter, we look at maintaining your financial independence and discuss ways that you can make your retirement profitable. There are activities that you can participate in that are low-impact and allow you to generate an income while you are enjoying your retirement. Let's take a look.

Chapter 6

MAINTAINING YOUR FINANCIAL INDEPENDENCE

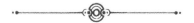

"Financial freedom is freedom from fear."
~ Robert Kiyosaki

T HE NATIONAL COUNCIL ON AGING (ncoa.org) shows that a staggering 16.5 million seniors living in America are not financially secure. Sadly, 64% of seniors rely on Social Security and Medicare to cover 90% of their daily needs. Even though they live above the federal poverty line, many seniors still struggle to make ends meet. Studies show that 47% of seniors over 50 do not have retirement savings, and about 50% are women. As alarming as this is, many seniors who do not plan for retirement are more likely to struggle with affording health care, living, and other necessary expenses like transportation, food, and medicine.

With the proper resources, knowledge, and trusted financial planners, you can plan to minimize future financial troubles, economic downturns, and inflation. Retiring comfortably would require you to have income-generating assets, 401K, IRA, life insurance, annuities, a lot of cash, bonds, or real estate.

You should know the exact number to retire comfortably and maintain financial independence. A great way to preserve your nest egg is to live below your needs and establish emergency fund accounts with other forms of income. Think creatively by asking yourself what you like to do for fun and how this can turn into income.

Activities to generate income for seniors

There are numerous activities that you can explore that can generate income. A side hustle is the new source of employment for many, where freelancing, providing services, or selling goods online can help create income. If you have invested in rental property or the stock market, you should have a passive income, but with the rising living costs, you might need more cash to secure yourself completely. Lucky for you, we are in a digital world, giving us the opportunity as seniors to earn additional income through tutoring, online classes, or freelancing. Whatever you decide to do, do enough research about the risks and rewards and commit to it. Here are some easy ways to generate income:

House-sit a neighbor's home or their pets

More people are traveling and need someone trustworthy to care for their pets and belongings. Consider checking online or advertising your services on your neighborhood's online pages or local newspapers. Doing this activity is a novelty, allowing you to change your environment by looking after someone's home or their beloved pets. Doing this for as little as a week allows you to change your daily routine. Your daily habits can become too consistent during retirement, but doing this activity can help reduce boredom. Especially if you live alone, the change of scenery could give you a new lease on life while providing help to someone who needs it. However, you want to make sure you are comfortable doing these positions.

Sell your unwanted goods

You could be sitting on a small fortune if you have spent much of your life working and buying little items for your home or lifestyle. You might have antique items, novelty items, or personal items that you have collected that could bring you extra money. The more antique the items are, the more valuable they could be. If you have anything that you feel is valuable, you can call a curator to inspect the items or research to determine the market value of those items. Websites like eBay allow you to sell items and earn money. However, you must factor in the shipping cost to determine whether the risk outweighs the reward. Yard or garage sales are other more practical ways to sell your items. You can get family members or trusted friends to help you keep things organized and sell your items for a fair price.

Tutor students

Many grade school students need assistance with school work, and parents often lack the time or expertise to tutor their children besides the popular subjects, like mathematics, English, and writing, which students may need. You can tutor students on playing an instrument if you have experience or teaching a language if you are bilingual. You could offer your services at local schools in the area, put up signs in libraries, or advertise online. You can choose to teach only one subject and one grade or work as a part-time substitute teacher. Tutoring can be flexible, and you can create a schedule on your terms. If you cannot drive to tutor the student, you can do 30-minute to 1-hour sessions online where you can tutor students using Zoom or Google Meet.

Sell your DIY projects

If you have taken up any hobbies like woodworking, art, or pottery, you can start a small online business selling the items you have made. This opportunity is great if you are not hurrying to generate an income and are looking for something to do with your time. You can get a web designer to create a website to advertise your work or ask local stores if they would like to stock your items and pay you a commission. You can ask a trusted loved one or friend about pricing your items. People enjoy buying popular homemade items: Christmas decorations, soaps, candles, or knitwear. Depending on the item, you can sell at farmer's markets, trade shows, or local community events. Another tip is to focus on having enough inventory to sell during the holiday season when people tend to buy more.

Sale your home-made baked goods

The scent of freshly baked chocolate chip cookies, especially from a seasoned baker, will create a long line of people eager to buy. You might not be able to indulge in sweet treats like before, but that shouldn't deter you from baking. First, decide what types of baked goods you want to prepare. Cookies, cupcakes, brownies, and candy are popular selling items, especially at farmer's markets, neighborhoods, and local events. To raise money for a particular cause, you can consider hosting a community bake sale. You can also sell baked goods at local businesses like hair salons, barber shops, etc. Also, consider taking special orders to sell more of your baked goods. Birthday parties are popular events where people may want to order homemade treats instead of getting the usual cakes and treats from grocery stores. This opportunity is excellent if you want to spend time doing something you love without over-exerting yourself.

Before selling baked goods, consider any specialty laws prohibiting you from selling. For instance, selling baked goods at farmer's markets will be under the Cottage Food Law. Be familiar with these laws, and ensure you do everything to keep yourself and others safe.

Explore freelancing opportunities

Thanks to the advancement of technology, you can gain access to freelancing opportunities available online. Of course, this will require you to be tech-savvy, but it is well worth it. A supplemented income is possible through doing online jobs. Websites like Fiverr and Upwork have made it easy for individuals who can use their skills and knowledge to help companies. These companies often look for anyone who can provide a quick return on a project like transcribing, ghostwriting, blogging, drawing, teaching, etc. When using sites like Fiverr and Upwork, the payments are safe and done through the site, so you can bid or search for projects that fit your capabilities. You will get paid through the site, so you don't have to manage to collect payments alone. Some popular services needed are writing memoirs, social media management, and virtual assistant. Anyone can turn their essential skills into a profitable service with some research and some learning. I highly recommend trying if you have experience and want to venture into freelancing. You can do it from the comfort of your home. All you need is a computer or laptop and a stable internet connection.

Become a ghostwriter

Becoming a ghostwriter can be challenging and fulfilling. It's a fun way to earn an income writing stories or books for small companies. If you are still getting familiar with this and want to learn more, a website like Udemy would be a great way to start. Websites like this offer short courses you can complete in a few weeks. Once you understand the requirements, you can use the credits in your portfolio. By the time you have collected enough credits, you can offer your services to other websites that need writers so you can get an idea of what you need to do as a ghostwriter. You can also increase job opportunities by showing potential clients your portfolio. The types of ghostwriting projects are limitless. You can write books, articles, website content, memoirs, and so much more. The only thing to remember is that the content will belong to the client, and your name won't be attached to the work. The client takes credit for your work, and you receive payment for your services.

You need to hone your skills and practice writing small pieces daily to strengthen your ability to understand assignments and type quickly and efficiently. Ghostwriters often work on strict time limits and must complete the assignment with spell checker and grammar checks, which takes practice. Tools such as Grammarly and the Hemingway app can help improve your grammar as you write. Here are a few tips to consider:

- **Familiarize yourself with the topic you will write about by reading and checking your facts.** If the client requires non-fiction work, you must ensure that the things you have written about are true. It can show bad form if there is nothing to connect your story to anything factual, and it can cost you, future clients.

- **Work on a writing sample portfolio.** Think about the kind of content you would like to write about and look for work online or in magazines that closely relate to what you would like to write about. Practice writing small pieces of 500 to 1000 words and perfect your spelling and grammar until you are confident.

- **Look for projects online where you can submit paid writing samples.** Typically, the client will require writing samples before hiring for a project. You can send your samples to them, but you should complete a paid writing sample.

Usually, paid writing samples are 1000 words or less, which may amount to up to $50. Doing a paid writing sample can help clients determine whether you are the right person for the job.

- **Consider attending writing conferences and networking events for writer groups in your area.** You can use social media to meet fellow writers and get advice on getting started with paying companies.

Be prepared and flexible enough to write about topics outside your comfort zone. You will need to research unfamiliar topics, complete your assignments timely, and present quality work. Overall, you can develop a steady source of income and become very profitable if you commit to it.

Start an online business

Although it may seem intimidating, you can sell anything online, from arts and crafts to 3rd-party manufactured items or your services. For small business owners, there are websites like Shopify, Amazon, and GoDaddy where you can sell items that generate a profit. If interested, look for courses to help you open an online shop. These courses focus on learning about the type of products to focus on selling so that you can generate positive revenue. It can be a long-term or short-term business, depending on your overall goals.

Thrift items for personal use or flip for profit

On Monday mornings, my community has heavy trash pick-up days where many discarded items are left on the curb. I drive around my neighborhood on Sundays to see what items can be refurbished, reused, or resold. On Sunday, while hunting for items, I came across an old grill in working condition that someone decided to put out as trash. It needed to be cleaned and a new propane tank to be as good as new, so I took it home and began working on it. The grill retailed for $300, and because I love to grill hamburgers, corn on the cob, and other meats, I found it to be a bargain. The cost to repair was under $50. Before using it, I needed to clean it up and fix bits and pieces. I found a lot of joy in the task, and once I could use it, I felt proud of my efforts. I had no intention of reselling the grill, but you could easily do the same with items you find that you may want to resell.

·You can use your online shop or local antique stores to resell any items you have found at second-hand stores like Goodwill or garage sales. For example, if you find an old painting that could be reused or resold, you could add a new frame, polish it, and load it on your online store or get a commission from local stores. The same goes for silverware, antiques, clothing, or jewelry.

I have an interesting story about heirlooms, antiques, and other valuables that I would like to share. In 2021, the oldest stamp in the world was discovered, which originated from British Guiana (now Guyana), a one-cent Magenta with a $10-15 million dollar valuation. A young boy found the piece of paper between his uncle's old valuables and sold it to a collector. Since that first resale, the value of the stamp has increased, and it has been sold again for an even higher price than before. The previous sale of the stamp was set at $9.48

million, but it has since increased in value as it is the oldest stamp in the world.

Money moves to master

Your first order of things when you try to master your money is to work on a budget. You need to consider the money that you have in your savings and the daily expenses you have. If there are any investments you would like to make, consider getting the help of a financial advisor to walk you through the process of acquisitions and explain the outcomes to you. Ensure you understand before you trust someone to help you invest in something that could hurt your financial security. Here are some creative ways in which you can obtain an income using your assets:

Reverse mortgage or refinance your home

Don't underestimate the asset you own—your home. Few people know how valuable their homes are and how you can use this asset to legally and ethically generate tax-free income. If you managed to pay off your mortgage and other debts, consider leveraging your home to generate an income. Any of these options and special programs offered through the federal government can help you without impacting your Social Security or Medicare benefits.

Did you know that you can use the home that you own to supplement your income?

A reverse mortgage is a loan for seniors to borrow against their home's equity. The great thing about this type of loan is that you receive tax-free payments from a lender, hence the name reverse mortgage. The caveat is that this loan must be paid back if you sell the property or when you pass on. The Home Equity Conversion Mortgages for Seniors is a federally backed program. Visit the HUD.Gov website to learn more if this option is for you.

If you want to improve your home's value, you can consider a home equity line of credit (HELOC). Qualifying for the HELOC will depend on your credit history, income, and home equity. Also, the types of HELOCs offered to you will vary from state to state, whether it be a fixed or variable interest rate attached to the loan. Typically, the HELOC is intended to be used to renovate a property to add more value to the property, but it's not limited to that. You can treat your HELOC as a checking account where you can withdraw amounts needed. However, consider this is still a loan, and your borrowed amount will accrue interest. With a HELOC, I renovated my home's kitchen and bathrooms. With the increased value of my home through renovating these rooms, I sold my home at a higher price and made a profit even after paying back the HELOC and interest.

Put your home on Airbnb

Are you considering downsizing your home? Whether you have too much house and live alone or with your spouse. If you intend to leave your home to your children once you pass on, consider leasing it. Airbnb is a popular way to rent your home short-term, which can generate a higher profit than renting long-term. You could even invest in a vacation home for the same purpose and use it occasionally, and when not in use, you can list it on Airbnb. It has become practically simple to put your home on Airbnb while having a 3rd party management company oversee everything, from cleaning to attending to the guests.

Dividend-stock options

If you have invested in the stock market, you can look at stock options that pay monthly dividends, which can supplement your income. Although investing in the stock market does impose risk, it can also generate wealth. The goal is to buy shares low and retain or sell shares higher than the original price you purchased for. You can choose to reinvest your dividends to purchase more shares. Buying shares weekly or monthly will help to increase the amount of shares you own. Do research on the companies you are interested in purchasing shares. If the company remains stable, you can be assured that your shares will earn profit. Some dividend stocks from popular and stable companies include Coca-Cola, Public Storage, Verizon Communications, Whirlpool Corp, and The Goldman Sachs Group Inc. Having a financial advisor to ask questions on investing and a certified public accountant about managing your financial portfolio and tax obligations is important.

Entrepreneurship for seniors

Your retirement is the ideal time to start that small business you have always dreamed of. You can take that step forward if your pension, savings, or other retirement accounts can assist you in your business's financial start-up and operating costs. Your business must be registered with the state and federal government for tax purposes. You will need an accountant, an attorney, and a banker. A great resource for small businesses in the United States is the Small Business Association (SBA).

Start to think of the type of business you would like to start. Find a gap or need in the market, and start a business that focuses on solving that need. I have a neighbor who opened a coffee shop. His idea was to have a gathering place where neighbors could walk from their houses with their dogs or bike there with their families. It was a charming shop with indoor and outdoor seating, the perfect place in the neighborhood to hang out.

Before you start, look at what you currently have and the necessary cost to get started. Write down the cost of supplies, equipment, and advertising. You could start your business at home, in a spare room you use as your office, or even your garage, which you use as a workshop. Let's say you want to make furniture like coffee tables or paint cabinets. You can start by cleaning out or organizing your garage to create enough room to work in your garage. This is a great way to save money rather than lease out a space to work. Once you have reached full capacity and your business is profitable, consider expanding.

It's important to be passionate about business and continually pour into it. Running a small business is hard work, and it requires the proper management of resources and energy to sustain it. Consider the stress and other physical exhaustion that comes with running a business. This is where delegation comes in. Hire the people who can help you with the day-to-day tasks, thus helping your business run more smoothly. You cannot do everything on your own; therefore, find the people you can hire to do the menial tasks so that you can focus on the more important roles you have in your business. This can include hiring someone to manage your website and social media accounts or an assistant who can manage your sales, orders, or deliveries.

Turning a passion project or a hobby into a business can be fun, but be aware of all the costs and requirements for legally running a business. You might enjoy doing something as a hobby but resent it when you run it as a business. A business is meant to create a profit, so consider being committed and having the correct mindset before deciding to run a business. Consider the financial implications and other important factors mentioned in this section.

Tax implications for seniors

As a senior, you will still be required to pay tax on any earnings you may incur. The great thing about that is the tax you pay depends on your specific income level. Understanding your tax obligations is vital; you may need professional assistance to work through your tax obligations. You may even be eligible for tax deductions or credits if you and your partner are over the age of 65 years, have a disability, or have a debilitating illness.

Tax credits for seniors

The list of tax credits you could qualify for as a senior is vast and beneficial, depending on your circumstances. A qualified tax professional or a reputable tax preparation software program can help determine what tax credits you may be eligible for. You could reduce your tax liability and identify potential credits and deductions, especially if you have a mortgage, business, or qualified medical expenses, which can maximize your savings.

If you have 401K or other pre-taxed retirement accounts, you will pay the taxes as you withdraw. While with Roth IRAs, if you have held your account for at least five years and at 59 and ½, you can withdraw earnings tax-free, without penalty.

Tax safety tips for seniors

A trusted certified public accountant (CPA) and a tax strategist are essential before tax filing. Laws and regulations are subject to change, so having a CPA and tax strategist can assist you with getting the tax credits and deductions you qualify for. Moreover, you must read everything you receive in the physical mailbox or email. Don't sign anything until you are sure of the source. Here are some tips to consider to keep you safe during tax season:

- Phone scammers are everywhere, and are likely to contact people to assist with taxes or even coerce them. They often pretend to be the IRS and threaten you with legal action if you do not settle your taxes immediately. You need to become familiar with IRS procedures and know which methods they use to contact you regarding your taxes. Note: The IRS will never call you; they will send a letter in the mail. If you do receive an IRS letter, contact your CPA.

- Your personal information is essential and needs to be protected at all times. Be wary of online scams that ask you to give your information to someone over the phone.

- Do not give your social security number or personal information to suspicious sources. Also, be suspicious of fake websites that pose as the US government website. Note: All federal government websites will have (.gov) and (http://).

- Ensure your computer is secure and the software is up to date. Also, ensure that your internet connection isn't being shared with anyone outside your home and that you have closed the site after completing your taxes online.

- Prevent identity theft and tax fraud by filing your taxes early or on time. The IRS will only accept returns filed only once to prevent fraud.

Basic financial literacy for seniors

Understanding the basics of finances and strategies to grow wealth is crucial. Many adults need to learn how investments work or how they can maximize their income once they have retired. There are simple ways to maintain a financial portfolio and improve your financial status. Still, it does require some fundamental knowledge. Knowing how to generate and grow money while saving and eliminating unnecessary expenses can help you in the long run.

- Set a budget and stick to it. It's helpful to track your expenses and know how much money to set aside each month. Keep a tab of your expenses and income and a list of things you would like to do in the future.

- Research or inquire about different retirement accounts and investment options. Speak to a financial advisor before you invest in anything. It is helpful to do so before you retire; some stern advice will help keep you from making wrong choices that will affect you in the long run.

- Take out the right insurance on your assets and invest in life insurance, disability insurance, and long-term care insurance to safeguard against any financial surprises.

- Pay any debt you have as quickly as possible, and consider debt consolidation to prevent an increase in interest rates.

- Pay attention to the news and stay updated with what's happening in the financial market. Seek the help of a financial advisor to help you understand any investments you have and how to keep them profitable.

- Check your credit with the three bureaus. You can

receive an annual free credit report from the three bureaus by law. Knowing what's on your credit report can help you prevent or protect yourself from fraud.

To successfully plan your retirement, you must understand how you will maintain your lifestyle. Consider your income, which can be from multiple sources such as social security benefits, pension, personal savings, retirement accounts, or a side hustle. You need to know how much money you anticipate to receive monthly and your tax liability. Being aware and prepared to enjoy your retirement comfortably without unnecessary stress is more rewarding.

Money-saving hacks for seniors

Being frugal once you retire can have many benefits. Having money in your account, not being a financial burden to your children, and being able to live out some of your dreams are only a few examples of those benefits. There is also the comfort of knowing you are prepared for any financial setbacks that may occur. Keeping track of your spending, whether with a financial planning app or writing it down in a journal, can help you keep track of your finances. Whatever you save can be grown through investments, which can be ideal if you plan to leave an inheritance for your benefactors.

As a senior, you want to be able to stretch your budget as much as you can. Consider the services you use, such as your telephone provider, and speak with customer service representatives at these companies. You could receive discount services or other loyalty rewards just for being a long-term customer.

Whether online or through advertisements, discover companies that offer discounted rates or services for seniors, whether dining out or purchasing household items. If you are a veteran, many places offer discounts to service members. Here are a few other money-saving hacks to consider:

- Get a low-interest credit card that offers cashback or other reward programs. Ensure you are spending below your limit, and pay off every month to avoid a dip in your credit score.

- Find coupons in newspapers, online, or in-store catalogs. These coupons can be very helpful for saving money on food or other necessary household items.

- Some communities or churches have food pantries where you can get staple food items donated from local grocery stores.

- Repurpose things you own instead of throwing them away and buying similar items.

- Save on electricity with solar light bulbs that recharge during the day and can be used at night.

- Shop at thrift stores.

- Get a library card instead of buying new books. You can also use your card to borrow DVDs or use a computer.

Alternatively, you could also cook more at home. Even if you are not a good cook, you can try new recipes you find online. This is an economical way to spend time with others and to enjoy a good meal with great company. It's less costly than going to a restaurant, and if you visit a different home each week, it will feel as exciting as going to a diner. Let's look at a few examples:

- Potlucks are a great example of this and could make for some interesting conversations if you add a theme. There are many fun ways you can organize gatherings.

- Consider cooking larger meals that you can freeze and reheat later. Curries and soups make great reheat options, and you can add fresh salads to the menu to add more variety to your meals.

- Ready-made pizzas and pies are affordable to eat at home because they take significantly less time to heat than cooking from scratch. They come in various flavors, and you can make it fun by designating a specific night of the week so that you don't exhaust yourself with different food options.

- Invest in a flask you can use for hot water if you love taking tea or coffee breaks. You can get one that has a slight tap to pour into your cup quickly and reuse it when you go camping or on long road trips.

If you love arts and crafts or other creative hobbies, join free groups in your community's recreation center, where the activities are free for seniors. It will be less costly than purchasing your equipment and supplies. My community has weekly events for seniors, including board game nights, bowling, and themed party nights.

You might not have control over every financial situation, but you can be prepared for it by saving money any way you can. Planning ahead, using free resources, and getting loyalty rewards and discounts are great places to start. Think of ways you can freely live your life while being affordable. In the next chapter, we'll look at making the ultimate bucket list. I had a lot of things I wanted to do when I retired, and having an ideal bucket list with milestones was a simple and straightforward approach to achieving my dream retirement. You, too, can follow your bucket list dreams with the tips from the next chapter and learn to live your best life with the right financial advice and the right way to follow your dreams. Let's go check it out.

Chapter 7

MAKING THE ULTIMATE BUCKET LIST

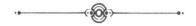

"You control your future, your destiny. What you think about comes about. By recording your dreams and goals on paper, you set in motion the process of becoming the person you most want to be. Put your future in good hands - your own."

~ Mark Victor Hansen

A STANFORD UNIVERSITY STUDY revealed that 78.5% of participants wanted to travel, which topped the list as the number one goal for their retirement. The desire to complete a plan was nearly tied to the desire to travel. Although the plans weren't specific, the study showed that making a plan specific to their goals was what they hoped to focus on in retirement. Interestingly, about 51% of participants desired to study or complete a degree. As you know, this study's results confirm that retirement is one of the peak times of life. Therefore, knowing life doesn't slow down once you retire shouldn't be a surprise.

A bucket list is something that we owe ourselves. It is the gift we give ourselves after achieving what we sought to do in our careers and with our families. It's a personal touch to living an entire life and completing monumental goals that say, " You did it!" You may want to travel to an exotic place or complete a project you might have started years ago, like writing a book. All it takes is one step forward and a little planning.

I wanted to do more with my life beyond my career, and at 55, I quit my director of sales position to focus on my passions. I wrote my goals on paper and began documenting when I reached a milestone. The most crucial thing to remember about creating a bucket list is that it's about you. You must add the things that will make you happy and mean the most to you.

How to start a bucket list

A bucket list can be adventurous or even very practical and straightforward. It could include doing something outside your comfort zone, like learning a new language or traveling to every US state. Your bucket list can be unique to you, or it can also include your spouse. There are so many fascinating things to do in this world, including exploring your neighborhood or places you have seen or learned about in movies or from others. Your bucket list is about creating and living an experience. To help you get started, here are seven questions to consider when creating your list:

1. What fun, unique, or interesting places do you hear about and desire to visit?

2. Is there a project you would like to do?

3. What is the most important goal you desire to achieve?

4. Are there milestones you have identified that can lead you to achieving your goal?

5. How can you prepare physically, mentally, and spiritually for the goals and plans you set for yourself?

6. Do you need support from a spouse, friend, or relative?

7. Does your goals and plans require thoughtful financial planning?

Your bucket list can be wild and crazy or simple and easy, but achievability is vital to cross it off the list. When you've established what you want to do most, choose the five to ten most achievable ones and work your way down your bucket list.

A bucket list can be intimidating if you have never considered it. Remember that you do not have to impress anyone with your plans. Think about general goals or even unrealistic ones. Make a list of all the things you can think of and choose which to prioritize. Once you have your list organized, you can work towards taking action. To sum up how you can start your bucket list, I have compiled a few tips to help you assemble your list:

1. Brainstorm your bucket list. Think of everything you have ever wanted to do, how achievable it is, and how likely you are to complete it. Consider whether your goals will affect your health and well-being and adjust them accordingly.

2. Itemize. Put the most important ones at the top of the list, but remember that this is not a set rule. If you want to start with smaller goals, add those to the list instead.

3. Get a calendar. Select a date and time to start your first item. Think of the resources you will need. Consider how much time it will take and if achieving it will be costly. Work your way around your goals if they are out of your financial reach. The aim is to have fun and accomplish your goals without putting yourself in distress.

4. Start working towards your goal and ask for help if needed. For example, if you want to travel to a new place, seek a travel consultant to help you with your hotel, airline, and leisure itineraries. If you desire to learn a new skill, join a beginner-friendly class so that you can learn fundamentals and create projects.

Benefits of having a bucket list

Creating a bucket list will be refreshing if you have lived a life confined by the rules of having a nine-to-five, raising kids, experiencing burnout, and following the usual life path. Completing a bucket list can be the first step to accessing your freedom through retirement. The list will help you to pay attention to your needs and the dreams you may have put on hold. Writing your goals down and putting them in a place where you can see them daily is a form of acknowledging them and putting effort into obtaining them. This doesn't mean you should abandon your responsibilities or throw caution to the wind. You should take the time during your retirement to consider what you would like to spend it best.

Your retirement is the ideal time to focus. Although you may be ready to start with your passion project or create plans, consider examining your financial and physical needs, as mentioned in previous chapters. Remember that you have time to focus on your long-term ambitions that give you a sense of purpose and fulfillment. Having a bucket list is about achieving contentment with what life has to offer.

As a bonus, you can include your spouse or family in some of your plans—such as seeing Yellowstone National Park or vacationing in Hawaii with your family. Now is a great time to make memories with the people you love by including them in the activities you have on your bucket list. Take the time to discuss your plans with your family, and ask them for their opinion about doing these plans together if you feel comfortable. You may be surprised to hear that your children desire to accompany you in your bucket list goals. You might even find that your partner has the same desires, and you can achieve them together.

Resources for creating your digital bucket list

There are endless possibilities when creating a bucket list. If you have a smartphone, computer, or tablet, many resources and apps are available to plan, organize, and keep track of your goals. There are apps and websites where you can subscribe to or become a member of. With many of these apps, whether on social media or in your local community app like NextDoor, you can easily connect with people with similar interests or ideas. Using apps is a great way to digitize your bucket list and keep track of your activities and experiences. Whether you want to learn how to ballroom dance or travel to different countries for cultural immersion, here are some free or affordable bucket list websites and apps you can try:

1. Travel Mapper

Although not necessarily a bucket list app, Travel Mapper is great for avid travelers who want to visit exciting places worldwide. This site is excellent for travel planning and budgeting, providing unique itineraries for getting the most out of your visit. Whether renting a bicycle to explore Copenhagen's historic sites or relaxing on the golden beaches in Australia, this site offers comprehensive and affordable travel planning to explore the city's best and most unique aspects of the country. Some of the features of this site include:

- Full daily itineraries to get the most out of your visits

- Map views of the region and directions for easier navigation

- Travel and budget tips

2. iWish

Organize your plans, find inspiration, and reflect on your goals in one place. Using this app helps create your ultimate wish list of over 1200 ideas to inspire your wellness, travel, financial, personal development, and more. What's great about this app is its functions that allow you to set and track your life goals. Some of the features are:

- Organize to-do lists

- Create vision boards, slideshows, or collages

- Track your progress and achievements

3. Soon

Soon is a unique social bucket list app that tracks your intended plans. This app lets you discover trending bucket list ideas and connect with your friends or loved ones. Features of this app include:

- Gain inspiration for bucket list ideas from other users

- Discover bucket list trends

- Receive reminders for your plans

4. Goal Setting Planner

To help you better plan your day-to-day and set goals, consider the Goal Setting Planner. This app helps you stay productive while achieving clarity and fulfillment. Some features of this app are:

- Daily task management of your SMART (specific, measurable, actionable, realistic, and timely) goals

- Notepad feature for documenting your questions, concerns, or thoughts

- Ability to share your goals with your support group, who can keep you accountable

Bucket list ideas to try

If you haven't been able to think about any ideas for your bucket list, here's some inspiration to help you get started:

1. Think about traveling to another state you have never been to but would like to go.

2. Take a class to learn a new language.

3. Go with your partner or friend on a road trip and spend the night at a place with a great view, excellent food options, and unique activities that are safe for seniors.

4. Spend time at the beach or rent a boat for a short sailing trip.

5. Go to a festival where you can spend a few days enjoying the company of others, making memories, and learning new experiences.

6. Offer your services as a volunteer at an animal shelter, a nursing home, or a community center. You don't have to do it full-time. Sign up for a month or two.

7. Visit some of the historical sites in the US that have significant meaning to the country's development.

8. Go on a safari.

9. Start blogging or write a memoir.

10. Enroll in a fitness program and commit to it for at least six weeks.

11. Start a small vegetable garden. You can grow things in pots or create a vertical garden if you don't have a backyard.

First and foremost, consider your health and safety, and select activities you feel comfortable doing. Consider your mindset before trying something new, and don't get discouraged if it doesn't work out how you desire. It's okay to put a little pressure on yourself, but do it without over-exerting yourself. Above all else, the fact that you considered and tried is all that matters.

Tips to conquer your bucket list

Now that we have established a bucket list, how to get started, and some ideas on what to do, let's look at how you can achieve these goals successfully.

1. Start small. Set achievable goals by starting small. Use a mind-mapping tool to break your bigger goals into smaller and achievable ones. For instance, if you desire to start your fitness journey, begin with a daily walk around your neighborhood or join a walking club.

2. Make your goals a priority. Use a daily planner or goal-setting apps to plan for your goals. Set the alarm to alert you to stay on track; this can help you focus and prioritize your goals.

3. Set SMART goals. Be specific about the goals you want to set. Make them achievable and realistic. Also, designate a time when you desire to achieve it.

4. Be open to the idea that your goals can change. Adjust them accordingly and work your way around them as you feel comfortable. It's a fun journey, so enjoy it.

Bucket list ideas for senior couples

During retirement, this is a time for you and your partner to enjoy each other's company and explore new experiences together. There are so many new experiences to behold; here are some ideas to consider:

1. Attend an opera. So many unique symphonies, ballets, and live theatre shows offer many unique experiences for couples. Over the years, I have developed a love for theatre, and it started with my spouse suggesting we attend a live show. We love dressing up and have suits and special attire dedicated to attending these performances. Even if you have never been to a live show, it's worth experiencing the variety of arts.

2. Take flight lessons. Have you ever desired to fly a plane? Consider taking introductory flight lessons taught by certified instructors to learn how to operate an aircraft. These lessons will consist of in-classroom coursework to understand how to fly a plane before actually flying the plane.

3. Enjoy a Michelin culinary experience. The Michelin Guide is the ultimate culinary experience guide to world-class restaurants. If you are a big foodie, like me, the best tacos, steakhouses, and more can be found in this guide. Use this guide to plan romantic date nights with your spouse in any city worldwide.

4. Take a cruise. For retirees who love to travel by sea, consider taking a cruise. Several cruise lines offer options more geared towards older adults than families with children. There are even cruise lines that can accommodate seniors with disabilities. You and your spouse can enjoy fine dining experiences, various amenities, and fun activities while at sea.

5. Explore a new scenery. You and your spouse can explore new sceneries near your home or take a few days off to explore a new city, state, or country. Learn something new about your hometown or the city where you live, and take pictures of how it looks now and compare it to how it looked before. If you are in a new place, talk with the locals, learn something new about the culture, collect a few souvenirs, and enjoy quality time with your spouse just living it up.

Money-saving bucket list ideas

1. Avoid paid subscriptions to apps, magazines, or memberships you don't actively use that incur a huge monthly expense.

2. Sign up for rebate apps, which give you cashback for groceries, gas, entertainment, and other items you purchase. Use your incentives to save for trips or fun activities on your bucket list.

3. Look in the newspaper or online for activities that you can do affordably.

4. Find promotional codes for cruise lines, airline tickets, hotels, and more, usually advertised online or through social media and travel newsletters.

5. Start a free Facebook group to connect with other retirees.

This chapter encourages you to live your life to the fullest. As a retiree, invest your time wisely in achieving your goals and living your dream retirement; that is what bucket lists are all about. Find your passions. Discover new experiences. Take the plunge, learn a new language, or visit the country you've always wanted to see. You only have one life, so be sure to live it to the fullest of your ability.

CONCLUSION

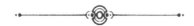

THIS GUIDE ON PLANNING your dream retirement has been one of the most meaningful projects I've completed. Writing this book has been an absolute joy because it gave me the time to think of how much I would like to help others and see my fellow retirees enjoy their golden years. It allowed me to reflect on the different things I did to make my retirement enjoyable and talk to you about ways you could avoid making some of my mistakes. It opened up conversations with my family and close friends and a new perspective on considering retirement as not the end but just the beginning.

For me, retiring was a tough choice because it was a step into the unknown, and although I had a plan, it was still a challenge. You might think retirement is about sleeping in and playing pickleball, but when that becomes boring, you need other ideas and plans to occupy your time.

You need a conclusive thought pattern on how you want to maximize your retirement. This includes thinking creatively about your finances to be in a better position to include activities you desire to do.

I want to convey how much fun retirement should be and that getting older doesn't have to mean not living a life full of excitement. There are many things that I have highlighted in each chapter to assist you with discovering new passions and deciding what's right for you. Each chapter covers a different need that I found helpful when putting together my plans and with tips like using apps and keeping a journal to set goals and manage my active schedule. These tips and ideas apply to anyone who has spent time thinking about their retirement and how to avoid anxiety over their finances and health.

Retirement should be a joyful and reflective time. Reflect on the tremendous opportunities in your life. You may have come to the end of your race in the corporate world, but that doesn't mean you have to stop running. Knowing how to make the most of your second chances in life should bring you peace and fulfillment.

Retirement does not mean giving up, but rather that you must slow down to enjoy the scenery and your time with friends and family. There are many ways to include your loved ones and friends in your plans.

Finally, each chapter contains fun ideas for making new memories. Think of this as the helping hand you can keep reaching for when you don't know what to do or need a fresh perspective on what you are currently doing. Whether joining a special group, learning a new skill, or starting a new business venture, this book guides you through tough decisions. It's here to help you figure out what you may have missed and how you can get back on track without giving up on the things you love. It's your guide, but mostly your friend on paper.

If anything, this guides you into spending more time doing what you have always dreamed of, like taking that trip or starting that hobby. It gives you the courage to ask those problematic financial questions and note the memories you are creating. Years from now, it can be the advice you can pass on to a loved one or friend experiencing the same feelings about their retirement. Best of all, you'll have more things to discuss that can bring you closer to living your best life.

Your golden years will be your most valuable, and planning your retirement and ensuring your stability in everything will bring you the fulfillment you need. Starting early with your finances is your first step. Knowing what you would like to do is your second step, and lastly, knowing how you want to do it will be the final step to a great retirement. Your happiness, health, and wellness are your most important goals.

My friend Pete reviewed this book with me while he was in the early stages of retirement. He knew what he wanted to do, but Pete still wondered how he would put it all together. His financial plans were set as I had helped him work through a few challenges, but once he got the idea of how he wanted to invest his time and energy, he was on his way. Pete and I go fishing from time to time as he found this to be his best pastime, and now and then, we get together with our family and friends and do a cookout or a potluck. Pete went from being always busy working and stressed to taking the time on a Sunday birding or spending time with his wife in their garden. His health improved, and he had more time to enjoy his family. He called this book life-changing, and I trust you will think the same. It can only get better from here on out.

This book is the start of you reaching your goals, so take action today. Take the first step to unlock a world of opportunities for your golden years. The sooner you start, the better the results. You can make things happen by remembering that every leap of faith begins with an idea, and every idea starts with a plan, so start your planning now!

If this book clarifies planning your retirement, then why not help someone else unlock the success of their retirement by leaving a review? I would love to hear how your life has changed and how I've helped you be a part of your successful retirement planning.

Made in the USA
Las Vegas, NV
24 May 2024

90322469R00085